THE COMPLETE LADY ERA GUIDE

The Complete Manual To Improve
Female Orgasm, Raise Low Libido,and
Address Female Sexual Dysfuntion

Dr. Chris David

Dr. Chris David

ABOUT THE BOOK

Lady Era was created to aid individuals with sexual issues and increase pleasure from sexual encounters. The Era pill, sometimes known as Viagra for women, is a novel medical medication developed as a women's libido medicine for people who want to enhance sexual arousal and experience pleasure during sexual activity. Scientists have recently used Sildenafil's beneficial medicinal characteristics to address issues specific to women. Women's Sildenafil has the same chemical composition as men's Viagra and acts via a similar mode of action, but it helps women boost their sensitivity to sexual stimulation in a way that male Viagra does not. Are you a woman looking for a pleasurable sexual experience, or a woman going through one that hurts?

CONTENTS

DR. CHRIS DAVID ERA

The Complete Lady Era Guide

The Complete Manual to Improve Female Orgasm, Raise Low Libido, and Address Female Sexual Dysfunction

TABLE OF CONTENTS

Is Lady Era influential? Lady Era: Is it Safe?

A short history about Lady Era

CHAPTER 1: WHAT YOU SHOULD KNOW ABOUT LADY ERA

What is Female Viagra?

What are the steps for obtaining them?

History of Female Viagra

How it all works in the Background

Medical Purposes

Other methods of treating female viagra

Are there any Libido-Enhancing Substances?

Summary

CHAPTER 2: WARNINGS AND PRECAUTIONS WOMEN WHO ARE UNABLE TO TAKE VIAGRA

What is Low Libido?

What is the Procedure for obtaining them?

History of Female Viagra

How it all works in the Background

Medical Purposes

Alternate Approaches

Are there any Libido-Enhancing Substances?

Summary

CHAPTER 2: WARNINGS AND PRECAUTIONS
Women who are unable to take Viagra

What is Low Libido?

Is Viagra an Effective Treatment for Lack of Sexual Desire in Women?

If a Lady Takes Viagra, what will happen to her? What are Some of the Possible Adverse Outcomes?

What May a Lady Take if She has Low Sex Desire Medication?

Osphena

Addyi

Vvleesi

CHAPTER 3: DOSAGES, MECHANISM OF ACTION AND SIDE EFFECTS

What is the Recommended Dosage of Viagra for Females? When it comes to Female Viagra, what's its functioning, and how secure is it?

In the battle between Addyi and Viagra drug

abuse is not permitted by label
The Goal and the Advantages

The Connected with the allowing cumatome

27% of sample Chapter 3: Dosages, Mechanism of Action and Side Effects

What is the Recommended Dosage of Viagra for Females? When it comes to Female Viagra, what's its functioning, and how secure is it?

In the battle between Addyi and Viagra drug abuse is not permitted by label The Goal and the Advantages

It's Connected with the Following Symptoms:

Flibanserin Mechanism of Action

Effectiveness of flibanserin

Menopausal Women are more Vulnerable to this Problem

Unwanted Results

Concerns Raised by the FDA Include the Following:

Notifications and Connections

Is Taking Viagra Everyday Good for You? Possible Substitutes for the Medicine Viagra
How long are the Effects Lasting?

Who Would Stand to Gain from this?

Biological

Psychological:

Consideration of cultural influences:

Side Effects

Addyi

Vyleesi

CHAPTER FOUR

COMBINATION WITH OTHER MEDICATIONS AND ALCOHOL

Avoiding Viagra in Specific Situations Consuming Nitrates

Viagra may interact with the following nitrates:

Suffering from Guanylate cyclase Deficiency The Combination of Viagra and Booze
Other Drugs and the Effects of Viagra

In-Depth Study of Drug Interactions

Inhibitors of PDE5

Sexual Dysfunction Medication

Antihypertensive Medications

A Small Number of Antifungal Medications

Viagra and other Drug Interactions

Supplements and Viagra

Herbs and Viagra

Viagra and Vitamins
Food and Viagra Interactions

Both Viagra and Vaccinations are now on the Market

Lab Testing and Viagra

THC and Cannabis Interactions with Viagra

Interactions between Viagra and certain Medical Conditions

Problems with the Liver or Kidneys

Problems with Bleeding

Cancers of the Blond

Deficiencies in Blood Cells

Risk of Heart Disease or Stroke

Problems with the Eyes

Risk of Heart Disease or Stroke

Ulcers in the Esophagus

Ashwagandha with Viagra: Do they Interact?

Is Viagra Safe to use with Statin Medications?

Are Viagra and Omeprazole Interfering with each other?

CHAPTER 5: BONUS CHAPTER: FREQUENTLY ASKED QUESTION

1. I'm Allergic to Claritin and Sudafed. Can I still Take Viagra? Do blood thinners like Warfarin or Xarelto interact with Viagra?

2. How long does Female Viagra need to start working?

3. Can you purchase Female Viagra without a medical prescription?

4. Are there alternatives to Female Viagra?

5. Is it possible to take Female Viagra for an 18-years-old girl?

6. Can Female Viagra be harmful?

7. Does Buspirone work the same way as Female Viagra?

8. Is Viagra Different for Men and Women?

9. What happens if a Transgender (Male to Female) takes Female Viagra?

10. What are the Medicines to raise Female Libido?

11. Can Male Viagra work on Females?

INTRODUCTION

Describe Lady Era.

In the pharmaceutical sector, Lady Era is advised to women who have decreased sex drive. The main ingredient that is active is sildenafil. Sildenafil is also present in Viagra, the most popular treatment for erectile dysfunction in men.

According to the manufacturer, this product is approved in some nations. In contrast, Lady Era is unavailable for purchase in the

UK. Since there isn't enough evidence to prove its effectiveness, it isn't yet licensed as a therapy for women with sexual dysfunction.

Is Lady Era a powerful woman?

In the United Kingdom, where it is not authorized for usage as a prescription, it has not been demonstrated that Lady Era is a successful treatment for female sexual dysfunction. Sildenafil, a main ingredient in Lady Era, has been investigated for its effect on female sexual dysfunction in a number of different research.

It has been demonstrated that sildenafil has no impact on women's sexual desire.

A smaller experiment with sildenafil for women with low sex drive revealed marginal improvement.

According to one study, sildenafil helps postmenopausal women's sex-related vaginal symptoms but not their desire for sex.

Sildenafil may mitigate the negative effects of SSRIs (antidepressants) on sexual function, according to a small study.

Question: is it safe?

Only when prescribed by a doctor are Lady Era and other sildenafil-containing medicines for female usage safe. This is not allowed in the UK, as was previously stated. Before giving the patient the drug, a thorough medical history would need to be taken to ensure there was no danger of harm.

Like sildenafil for men, it's possible that Lady Era will have just as many negative effects on women as they do on men. Due to its lack of strict regulation, it is also unknown if Lady Era contains what it claims to or if there are dangerous dosages of medication.

According to an unbiased investigation by the Therapeutic Goods Administration, Lady Era contains a number of chemicals that the manufacturers have not disclosed.

A SHORT HISTORY OF LADY ERA

Researchers think Lady Era helps men achieve better erections similarly to Viagra because it has the same active ingredient as Viagra (Sildenafil). However, it might also increase a woman's sex arousal.

Surveys on the efficacy of Lady Era produced a range of findings. It's debatable if it arouses sexual desire or not. Others disagree with those who claim it does.

Both men and women experience symptoms like dizziness frequently. Even though the risks outweigh the advantages for the majority of women, the medication is still not approved in the United Kingdom.

CHAPTER ONE

THE LADY ERA: WHAT YOU NEED TO KNOW

How does female Viagra work?

An Overview of Female Viagra

For a lot of women, their sexual desire changes over the course of their life, frequently as a result of strain, changes in their intimate relationships, and hormonal problems like pregnancy and anovulation. 10% of women, however, experience low levels of sex drive. The term used by doctors to describe this illness is hypoactive sexual desire disorder (HSDD).

A few over-the-counter supplements can be used to treat the issue, but their effectiveness is limited and largely unproven. In the recent years, the FDA has approved two brand-new prescription medications to treat HSDD. The colloquial name for these therapies—"Female Viagra"—is a reference to the drug men can start taking for sex-related problems. There is no denying that men with "plumbing problems" can benefit from using Viagra. Viagra and other related medications can be helpful when a man struggles to achieve or maintain an erection that is strong enough to engage in sex. These men frequently still yearn for sex but are unable to trigger a biological response in their bodies when they want to engage in it. The medications increase blood flow and relax the genital tissues, which results in an erection.

The problem of low libido in women is more complex.

As a result, we are treating HSDD, which requires a more specialised approach.

Medications, two.

The following therapies are FDA-approved for treating HSDD:

- Flibanserin (Addyi) is a tablet that you take at night.
- Bremelanotide (Vyleesi) injections are given 45 minutes prior to sexual activity.

Doctors advise getting no more than eight shots every month, and they should be spaced 24 hours apart.

What steps are involved in getting female viagra?

The phrase "female Viagra" is frequently used in slang to describe drugs intended to treat female sexual dysfunction, especially those that attempt to raise arousal or desire. Flibanserin (Addyi) and bremelanotide (Vyleesi) are two drugs for this use that the FDA has approved. An overview of how to take these drugs is provided below:

1. Flibanserin (Addy)

Flibanserin must be prescribed by a healthcare professional who can assess your unique needs and hazards in order to be obtained.

Dosage: A 100 mg tablet taken once day at bedtime is the usual dosage advice. It's crucial to adhere to the dose recommendations made by your doctor.

Flibanserin should be taken consistently, and it can take a few weeks before you see an improvement in your arousal or sexual desire.

Alcohol Use: It's important to abstain from alcohol while taking flibanserin because it can cause low blood pressure and fainting.

Dizziness, nauseousness, and tiredness are examples of frequent adverse effects. Consult a medical professional if you develop any severe or worrisome side effects.

2. Bremelanotide (Vyleesi)

Bremelanotide is only available with a prescription from a healthcare professional, just like flibanserin.

Use of an autoinjector pen is required to administer bremelanotide as a subcutaneous injection (under the skin). You will receive instructions from your healthcare practitioner on how to use it, and you should carefully heed their advice.

Timing: At least 45 minutes before planned sexual activity, the injection is often given.

Bremelanotide should not be used more than once every 24 hours or more frequently than eight times per month.

Typical side effects may include headache, flushing, and nausea. Consult your healthcare practitioner if you develop severe or out of the ordinary adverse effects.

Note: It's crucial to keep in mind that these drugs may or may not work for each individual patient, and their efficacy can vary. Additionally, treating female sexual dysfunction frequently necessitates a multifaceted strategy that may include therapy, way of life adjustments, and dealing with underlying medical or psychological issues.

It's critical to have an honest discussion with a licenced healthcare provider before considering the usage of any drug to treat sexual dysfunction. To protect your safety and wellbeing, they can evaluate your particular needs, offer advice on possible treatment options, and keep track of your development.

As they may cause negative effects and interact with other medications or medical conditions, these medications should not be used without a prescription or without first visiting a healthcare provider.

HISTORY OF FEMALE VIAGRA

When pharmaceutical companies started looking at possible treatments for female sexual dysfunction (FSD), the idea of a "female Viagra" attracted a lot of attention in the late 1990s and early 2000s. Low sexual desire, difficulty being aroused, and difficulties eliciting orgasm are just a few of the problems covered by FSD.

Flibanserin was one of the first drugs to come under consideration as a possible female version of Viagra. Although initially intended to treat depression, flobanserin only had a limited amount of success in that regard. It was noted that it may, in some women, increase sexual desire. Later, the medication was changed to treat premenopausal women with hypoactive sexual desire disorder (HSDD).

The U.S. Food and Drug Administration (FDA) authorised flibanserin, sold under the trade name "Addyi," in August 2015 as the first medicine especially made to treat HSDD in women. It functions by having an impact on specific neurotransmitters in the brain. Due of worries about its effectiveness and adverse effects, it has encountered significant criticism and had only limited success.

The FDA authorised bremelanotide, a drug marketed under the trade name "Vyleesi," in June 2019. For the treatment of acquired, generalised hypoactive sexual desire disorder (HSDD) in premenopausal women, bremelanotide is administered intravenously. It functions by boosting blood flow to the vaginal region and turning on specific brain receptors.

Both the prescription drugs flibanserin and bremelanotide have undesirable side effects. When it comes to mechanism or effectiveness, they are not comparable to Viagra. Research into effective treatments for female sex dysfunction is still ongoing, and the field is constantly changing due to new discoveries and potential medications.

It's crucial for women who are experiencing sexual dysfunction to speak with medical experts about their concerns and look into the best course of treatment, which may entail medication, therapy, lifestyle changes, or a combination of these. The history of "female Viagra" demonstrates how difficult it is to treat female sexual dysfunction and how difficult it is to create successful treatments.

background information on how female Viagra functions
In particular, the mechanisms by which medications like flibanserin (Addyi) and bremelanotide (Vyleesi) treat hypoactive sexual desire disorder (HSDD) in females are complicated and poorly understood. These medications focus on various pathways that govern a woman's sexual response and desire. An outline of their background operations is provided below:

Flibanserin (Addyi)

- Flibanserin primarily affects serotonin receptors in the brain by acting as an agonist and antagonist of serotonin receptors, which regulates serotonin and dopamine. It modifies dopamine and serotonin activity in specific regions of the brain connected to arousal and sexual desire.
- Neurotransmitter Rebalancing: It is thought that flibanserin functions by restoring a healthy balance among these neurotransmitters, which have been linked to the control of sexual desire.

- Long-Term Use: Flibanserin is taken consistently over a long period of time, and it may take a few weeks before its effectiveness is felt. It aims to address premenopausal women's persistent lack of sexual desire.

It's important to proceed cautiously when considering claims that certain drugs or products will increase libido or sexual desire. These substances' efficacy and safety can differ greatly, and some may have unfavourable side effects or interact with prescription drugs you might be taking. Before attempting any libido-enhancing substances, it's also very important to speak with a medical professional, especially if you have underlying medical conditions or are taking medication.

The following medications have been linked to potential libido-boosting effects, though their efficacy and safety can differ:

Aphrodisiac Foods: Oysters, chocolate, and a few spices are among the foods thought to have aphrodisiac effects. Although these foods may be linked to sensual or romantic experiences, their actual effects on libido is often anecdotal Bremelanotide (Vyleesi) :

- Bremelanotide activates melanocortin receptors in the brain, specifically the MC4 receptor, by acting as a non-selective agonist. The control of sexual arousal and desire is mediated by these receptors.
- Blood Flow: Bremelanotide also improves blood flow to the genital area, which may help to arouse sexual desire.
- Rapid Onset: Bremelanotide is given as needed, usually 45 minutes prior to sexual activity, unlike flibanserin. When used as prescribed, it seeks to improve arousal and desire for sexual activity more quickly.

It's crucial to understand that these drugs don't function the same way that sildenafil (Viagra), a drug used to treat erectile dysfunction in men, does. Drugs for male erectile dysfunction mainly function by boosting blood flow to the penis, which facilitates an erection. A more intricate interplay of psychological, hormonal, and neurological factors affects female sexual desire and arousal.

Female Viagra for medical purposes

1. Hypoactive Sexual Desire Disorder (HSDD) treatment:
   - For the treatment of HSDD in premenopausal women, flibanserin (Addyi) and bremelanotide (Vyleesi) are approved medications. A persistent and distressing

lack of sexual desire or interest that results in emotional distress or interpersonal difficulties is a hallmark of HSDD.

- Recognised as a medical condition, HSDD can have a detrimental effect on a person's general health and quality of life. It is a chronic and uncomfortable condition rather than merely an issue of infrequently having little sexual desire.

2. Enhanced sexual arousal and desire:

- The goal of flibanserin (Addyi) is to increase sexual desire in HSDD-affected women who have low libido levels. It helps to boost sexual interest by working on specific neurotransmitters in the brain.
- In order to increase sexual desire and arousal in females with acquired, generalised HSDD, bremelanotide (Vyleesi) is prescribed. The brain's melanocortin receptors are primarily activated by it.

It's critical to stress that these drugs are not equivalent to "Viagra" for men and are not meant for recreational or casual use. The use of these medications should be supported by a thorough assessment by a licenced healthcare professional and a confirmation of HSDD.

Other methods of treating Female Vigra

1. Counselling and Therapy

In order to address the psychological and emotional aspects of sexual dysfunction, such as relationship problems, stress, anxiety, and body image issues, sex therapy or couples therapy can be very effective.

People can recognise and alter unfavourable thought and behaviour patterns in relation to sex and intimacy with the aid of cognitive-behavioral therapy (CBT).

2. Changes in Personality:

- Regular exercise may increase sexual desire and function while also enhancing general well-being.
- Anxiety about sexual performance can be lessened by practising relaxation strategies, being mindful, or engaging in meditation.
- The overall physical and mental health, which can impact sexual well-being, can be improved with a healthy diet and enough sleep.

3. Education and Communication

- Improved sexual satisfaction and intimacy can result from open and honest communication about needs, wants, and concerns with a partner.
- Individuals who receive sexual education and information may feel less anxious and more confident as they gain a better understanding of their bodies and sexual responses.

4. **Hormone Treatment:** Hormonal imbalances, such as those brought on by menopause, can sometimes be a factor in sexual dysfunction in women. Under the direction of a healthcare professional, hormone replacement therapy (HRT) may be taken into consideration.

5. **Pelvic Floor Rehabilitation:** Physical therapy for the pelvic floor may help women who feel pain or discomfort during sex. Issues with relaxation and muscle tension can be helped by a qualified therapist.

6. **Sensate Focus Training**: These sex therapy exercises, which frequently involve non-genital touching and exploration, are

meant to improve comfort and intimacy between partners.

7. **Over-the-Counter Items**: Using over-the-counter lubricants or moisturisers made specifically for sexual use, some people find relief from sexual discomfort or dryness. These items can improve comfort while engaging in sexual activity.

8. **Body-Mind Techniques**: Yoga, tantra, and mindfulness techniques can help people relax, become more aware of their bodies, and connect emotionally, all of which can have a positive impact on their sexual experiences.

9. **Various Treatments**: For possible sexual enhancement, some people look into herbal supplements like ginseng or maca root. The effectiveness and safety of these products, however, are not well established.

Different Libido-Enhancing Substance

It's important to proceed cautiously when considering claims that certain drugs or products will increase libido or sexual desire. These substances' efficacy and safety can differ greatly, and some may have unfavourable side effects or interact with prescription drugs you might be taking. Before attempting any libido-enhancing substances, it's also very important to speak with a medical professional, especially if you have underlying medical conditions or are taking medication.

The following medications have been linked to potential libido-boosting effects, though their efficacy and safety can differ:

Aphrodisiac Foods: Oysters, chocolate, and a few spices are among the foods thought to have aphrodisiac effects. Although these foods may be linked to sensual or romantic experiences, their actual effects on libido is often anecdotal.

Herbal supplements: In the past, people have used specific herbs and herbal supplements to increase libido. Ginseng, maca root, and horny goat weed are a few examples. Although some people claim that these herbs have beneficial effects, there is not much scientific evidence to back this up.

Factors related to lifestyle: Libido can be significantly increased by leading a healthy lifestyle. A healthy sex drive can be influenced by regular exercise, a balanced diet, stress reduction, and enough sleep.

Pharmaceuticals: To treat particular sexual dysfunction issues, medical professionals may occasionally prescribe drugs like sildenafil (Viagra) or flibanserin (Addyi). Only a healthcare professional should be consulted when taking these medications.

Psychological counselling: Stress, anxiety, and other psychological issues are frequently connected to low libido or low sexual desire. or problems in relationships. Counselling or therapy may be more beneficial in these situations than any drug or medication.

Hormone Therapy: To treat low libido in some people with hormonal imbalances, hormone replacement therapy may be advised. Only a healthcare professional should direct you in doing this.

Remember that there is no one-size-fits-all approach to libido enhancement and that what works for one person might not work for another. In addition, there may be a lack of scientific evidence to back up the claims made by some substances marketed as libido boosters, and their safety may not be well established.

It is advised to speak with a healthcare provider before using any medication or treatment to boost libido. This person can help determine the underlying causes of any libido-related issues and offer advice and suggestions tailored to your unique health and situation. Additionally, they can aid you in making decisions about any potential treatments or dietary supplements.

CHAPTER TWO

Flibanserin (Female Viagra - Addyi) Warnings and Precautions

Flibanserin, sold under the trade name Addyi, is a drug used to treat hypoactive sexual desire disorder (HSDD), which causes premenopausal women to have low levels of sex desire. While it may work for some women, there are a number of warnings and precautions that need to be taken into account before use. We go into more detail about these cautions and warnings below:

Boxed Caution:

The most serious type of warning issued by the U.S. Food and Drug Administration (FDA) is the Boxed Warning, also known as a Black Box Warning, which is present on flibanserin. The warning emphasises the danger of syncope (fainting) and severe hypotension (low blood pressure) when taking Addyi, especially when combined with alcohol.

Secondly, Restricted Distribution Under the FDA's Risk Evaluation and Mitigation Strategy (REMS) programme, Addyi is only accessible through a limited programme.

This is due to the significant risks involved in using it.

3. Inhibitory conditions:

The following circumstances are examples of when Addyi should not be used:

Alcohol: It shouldn't be taken with alcohol because doing so can have serious negative effects, including fainting and a significant drop in blood pressure.

Hepatic Impairment: Addyi should be avoided by patients with liver impairment as it may increase drug exposure and the possibility of negative side effects.

When combined with potent CYP3A4 Inhibitors: Due to the possibility of elevated flibanserin levels and negative effects, concurrent use with potent CYP3A4 inhibitors (like ketoconazole or ritonavir) is not advised.

4. Drinking alcohol

Alcohol should be completely avoided by patients both while taking Addyi and for at least two days (48 hours) after stopping the medication. Syncope and severe hypotension risks can both be increased by alcohol.

5. Syncope and Hypotension Risk:

A significant drop in blood pressure from flibanserin may result in fainting. Patients should be informed of the risk and advised to refrain from tasks that call for alertness (such as operating heavy machinery) until they are familiar with how Addyi affects them.

Central Nervous System (CNS) Effects

Driving or performing other tasks that call for mental alertness may become difficult while taking Addyi because of somnolence (drowsiness) and sedation. While feeling these effects, patients should refrain from risky activities.

7. Potential Connections

Flibanserin can interact with a number of drugs, including potent CYP3A4 inhibitors, which may raise blood levels and increase the possibility of negative effects. Patients should disclose all medications they are taking to their healthcare provider.

8. Nursing and pregnancy:

Addyi's effectiveness and safety during pregnancy and breast-feeding have not been proven. In these populations, it should be used with caution, and the potential advantages and risks should be carefully weighed.

9. Variations in Heart Rate and Blood Pressure:

Blood pressure and heart rate may slightly increase as a result of flibanserin. The medication should be used with caution by patients who have cardiovascular conditions, and these parameters should be watched for changes.

10. Discontinuation: Patients should be instructed on how to stop taking Addyi safely, and medical professionals should be alert to any possible withdrawal symptoms or changes in sexual desire that might appear after stopping.

11. Patient Education: Patients should be given comprehensive information about the dangers and safety measures related to Addyi, and they should be encouraged to ask questions and get clarification from their healthcare provider.

In conclusion, Flibanserin (Addyi), also known as "Female Viagra," is a drug that has been given the go-ahead to treat HSDD in premenopausal women. However, using it carries serious risks, including the possibility of syncope, severe hypotension, and interactions with certain drugs and alcohol. Patients who are thinking about taking Addyi should have a thorough conversation with their doctor to weigh the potential advantages and risks and make sure it is the best course of action for their particular situation. It is essential to adhere to all medical advice.

What causes a low libido? Low sexual desire or libido is a common issue that can affect both men and women. Low libido can have a wide range of possible causes that differ from person to person. We will examine a variety of causes of low libido in this thorough overview, including psychological, physical, and relationship-related issues.

Physical causes include:

Hormonal Imbalances: Sexual desire is strongly influenced by hormones. Reduced libido may be caused by hormonal imbalances involving thyroid hormones, oestrogen, and testosterone (in both men and women).

Medication: Some antidepressants, antihypertensives, and antipsychotics can have unwanted side effects that lower sexual desire.

Medical Conditions: A number of medical issues, such as long-term conditions like diabetes, heart disease, and cancer, as well as conditions that affect the reproductive system, such as erectile dysfunction (ED) and polycystic ovary syndrome (PCOS).

Ageing and Menopause: In women, the hormonal changes brought on by menopause may cause a decrease in sexual desire. Age-related declines in testosterone in men can also result in decreased libido.

2. Causes that are psychological

Stress: Excessive stress, whether it be from work, money, or personal matters, can lessen sexual desire. The body's reaction to stress frequently inhibits the production of sex hormones.

Depression and Anxiety: Mental health issues like depression and anxiety can cause a low libido. Some of the drugs prescribed to treat these conditions may also have adverse effects on the sex life.

Body Image Problems: Sexual desire can be impacted by poor self-esteem and a negative body image. discomfort or dissatisfaction with one's Reduced interest in sexual activity due to appearance.

Sexual trauma or past abuse: These experiences can have a lasting impact on one's sexual desire and may cause one to avoid engaging in sexual activity.

3. Causes in Relationships: Low libido can be caused by communication problems, unresolved conflicts, or a lack of emotional connection with a partner.

Relationship Issues: Consistent relationship problems, like infidelity, trust issues, or a lack of emotional intimacy, can diminish sexual desire.

Partner's Sexual Dysfunction: Sexual dysfunction in a partner, such as ED or early ejaculation, can reduce libido and have an impact on both partners' satisfaction in a sexual relationship.

Boredom or Routine: A lack of novelty and excitement in the relationship or monotony in sexual routines can reduce sexual desire long term.

4. Behavioural and Lifestyle Factors:

Poor Sleep: Lack of sleep, fatigue, and reduced energy can all affect one's desire to engage in sexual activity.

Unhealthy lifestyle practises: Sedentary living, drinking too much alcohol, and smoking can all have a negative effect on libido.

Diet and nutrition: Sexual function and general health can be impacted by a diet that is inadequate in essential nutrients.

Lack of Physical Activity: Regular exercise improves blood flow, energy levels, and mood, all of which have a positive impact on libido.

Substance Abuse: Abuse of prescription drugs or illicit drugs can cause a decline in sexual interest.

4. Social and Cultural Aspects:

Cultural and Religious Beliefs: A person's cultural or religious background and beliefs may have an impact on how they view sex and their desire for it.

societal influences, including an individual's sexual desire and self-perception can be significantly impacted by sexual harassment, gender-based violence, or societal stigmas surrounding sexuality.

Personal Principles and Values:

Personal Values: One's sexual desire may be influenced by their personal sexual values and beliefs. An individual with conservative values, for instance, might feel guilty or ashamed about having sexual desires.

Perspectives on Sexuality: Libido can be affected by individual sexual attitudes, such as being honest and accepting of one's own desires.

In conclusion, a low libido can result from a number of factors, including lifestyle, relationship-related, psychological, and physical factors. It is important to understand that low libido is a problem that affects many people and that it can frequently be resolved through communication, lifestyle adjustments, medical interventions, or counselling. If having a low libido bothers you or has an impact on your quality of life, consulting a medical expert or therapist can help in figuring out the root causes and creating a unique treatment plan to deal with the problem. Navigating and resolving any relationship-related issues causing low libido also requires open and honest communication with a partner.

Is Viagra a successful treatment for female insecurities about sex?

Viagra (sildenafil) is a drug used to treat erectile dysfunction (ED) in men. It does this by boosting blood flow to the penis, making it easier to achieve and maintain an erection. It is not intended for use in women to address sex insecurities or to increase sexual desire, nor has it received regulatory authority's approval in this regard.

However, there are a number of crucial factors to take into account when talking about the potential use of Viagra or comparable drugs in women and the bigger picture of addressing sexual insecurities:

1. Viagra's Action Mechanism

Viagra works by blocking the phosphodiesterase type 5 (PDE5) enzyme, which causes the blood vessels in the penis to relax and flow more freely. The male anatomy is unique to this mechanism, which has no immediate effects.

2. Women's Products Lack FDA Approval:

Viagra has not been given FDA (Food and Drug

Administration) approval for use in females. Other drugs for female sexual dysfunction have received FDA approval, including flibanserin (Addyi) and bremelanotide (Vyleesi), which target various aspects of female sexual function, specifically addressing low sexual desire (Hypoactive Sexual Desire Disorder or HSDD) and sexual arousal problems, respectively.

3. Dealing with Women's Sexual Insecurities

Sexual insecurities in women can be caused by a variety of things, such as psychological, emotional, and relationship problems. Despite the fact that drugs like Viagra may not be directly helpful, treating these insecurities frequently necessitates a more all-encompassing strategy that may include therapy, partner communication, and enhancing self-esteem and body image.

4. The Function of Therapy and Communication

Honest and upfront Intimacy can be increased and sexrelated insecurities can be addressed through communication with a partner. Many women discover that communicating their preferences, worries, and desires to their partner can result in a more fulfilling sexual connection.

To address sexual insecurities, psychotherapy or counselling, including individual and couple's therapy, can be very helpful. Therapists can offer strategies for boosting confidence and enhancing sexual satisfaction as well as assist people in exploring and understanding the underlying causes of their insecurities.

5. Drugs Suitable for Women:

The FDA has given the drugs libanserin (Addyi) and bremelanotide (Vyleesi) approval to treat particular aspects of female sexual dysfunction. While Vyleesi is used to treat premenopausal women with acquired, generalised hypoactive sexual desire disorder (HSDD), Addyi is meant to treat low sexual desire (HSDD). In contrast to Viagra, these drugs target specific neurotransmitters and receptors in the brain to arouse or increase sexual desire in females.

6. Dangers and negative effects:

Like all medicines, Viagra has potential risks and side effects, and these may be different for men and women. The lack of safety and efficacy information for this population makes it unwise for women to use Viagra.

Any sexual health issues or insecurities must be discussed with a healthcare professional because self-medicating with drugs not approved for your particular condition can be risky and may not adequately address the underlying problems.

In conclusion, Viagra is not an approved or advised treatment for treating female sex insecurities or enhancing female sexual desire. Sexual reticence Often involving emotional, psychological, and relational factors, they are complex and multifaceted in women. For these insecurities to be addressed, it may be necessary to communicate, engage in therapy, and occasionally take drugs that are especially formulated and approved for female sexual dysfunction. In order to address sexual concerns and enhance overall sexual satisfaction in women, it is crucial to speak with a healthcare professional or therapist.

What will happen to a woman who takes Viagra? What are a few potential negative effects?

Men with erectile dysfunction (ED) can be treated with the aid of the drug Viagra (sildenafil). It functions by boosting blood flow to the penis, which makes getting and keeping an erection easier. Although women are not permitted to use Viagra, some may wonder what would happen if they did and what risks or adverse effects might occur.

It's important to stress that Viagra is not meant to be used by women, and the discussion that follows is solely for informational purposes. Any woman considering Viagra or dealing with erectile dysfunction should speak with a healthcare professional for an accurate assessment and advice catered to her individual needs.

Here are some details on possible outcomes if a woman takes Viagra and possibly harmful outcomes

Possibly Adverse Effects of Female Viagra Use:

Similar to how it affects men, Viagra may cause increased blood flow in a woman's genital region. This could result in increased sensitivity and engorgement of the clitoris and vaginal tissues. Some women might interpret this as increased responsiveness or arousal for sexual purposes.

Potential for Improved Natural Lubrication: Improved natural lubrication in the vaginal area may result from increased blood flow, which could make sexual activity more comfortable.

Placebo Effect: When taking Viagra, some women might experience increased sexual satisfaction as a result of a placebo effect. Sexual function may improve if a patient believes their medication is working.

Possible Viagra side effects in women:

Limited Evidence: One of the key problems with the There is little scientific evidence that Viagra is effective and safe for treating female erectile dysfunction in women. There is a dearth of thorough information on how Viagra affects women, with the majority of clinical trials and research on the subject concentrating on men.

Side Effects: Although the likelihood and severity of side effects may vary, women taking Viagra may experience side effects that are similar to those experienced by men.
The following are some typical Viagra side effects:

Headache

Flushing (warmth and redness in the upper body and face) uneasy stomach nasal clogging Dizziness visual disturbances (including modifications to colour perception)

Cardiovascular Effects: Viagra may have an impact on blood pressure, raising questions about possible cardiovascular side effects in female users. It may occasionally result in a a drop in blood pressure that causes lightheadedness or fainting. Women who have had cardiovascular problems in the past or who take drugs that affect blood pressure should use caution.

Sexual dysfunction in women is frequently caused by hormonal and psychological issues, such as low sexual desire (also known as hyperactive sexual desire disorder, or HSDD). Viagra does not address these issues. Different aspects of sexual response are targeted by other drugs, including flibanserin (Addyi) and bremelanotide (Vyleesi), which are specifically approved for treating female sexual dysfunction.

Unknown Long-Term Effects: Because most studies have been short-term and have focused on men, it is unclear what the long-term effects of Viagra use in women will be.

Viagra is not advised for use during pregnancy or while nursing because there are safety concerns. Women ought to When breastfeeding or pregnant, stay away from Viagra.

Conclusion:

Viagra is a medication used to treat erectile dysfunction in men; regulatory bodies neither recommend nor approve its use in women. While some female sexual dysfunction sufferers may take Viagra and feel lubricated, their blood flow may increase, or they may experience a placebo effect, Viagra's effectiveness and safety are not wellestablished. Additionally, it's important to consider any possible side effects and cardiovascular issues.

Women should seek advice from a healthcare professional if they are experiencing sexual dysfunction or have concerns about their sexual health. Healthcare professionals can assist in choosing the best course of action based on specific needs and circumstances. Additional treatment options that are intended and approved for treating female sexual dysfunction are also available. Open Addressing sexual health issues safely and effectively requires communication with a healthcare professional.

What Medications Can a Woman Take if She Has Low Sex Desire?

Low sexual desire, also referred to as Hypoactive Sexual Desire Disorder (HSDD), can have a serious negative effect on a woman's relationships and quality of life. Thankfully, a number of drugs have been created to treat this issue and aid women in regaining their sexual desire and satisfaction. In this article, we'll look at a few of the drugs a woman might want to think about if her sex desire is low.

First, libanserin (Addyi)

The U.S. Food and Drug Administration (FDA) has only recently approved the use of flibanserin to treat HSDD in premenopausal women. It is sold under the Addyi brand name.

Flibanserin affects the brain's neurotransmitters in a way that specifically targets serotonin and dopamine levels. By restoring the balance of these chemicals, it is thought to increase sexual desire.

Administration and Dosage: The suggested Time is Taking 100 mg at nighttime is the recommended dosage.

Effectiveness: According to clinical trials, women who took Addyi had a modestly higher sex desire than women who took a placebo. Although it may not be helpful for all HSDD sufferers, the improvement's magnitude is thought to be moderate.

Side Effects: Common side effects include drowsiness, nausea, dry mouth, fatigue, and somnolence. A dangerous drop in blood pressure and fainting might result from its interactions with alcohol and some medicines.

Bremelanotide (Vyleesi), : Another medication approved by the FDA for the treatment of HSDD in premenopausal women is bremelanotide, which is sold under the trade name Vyleesi.

Efficacy Mechanism: Bremelanotide is a central nervous system-active melanocortin receptor agonist increased sexual desire due to the nervous system.

Dosage and Administration: It is given as a subcutaneous (under the skin) self-injection at least 45 minutes before planned sexual activity.

Effectiveness: According to clinical trials, women who received bremelanotide reported slightly higher levels of sexual desire and more satisfying sexual experiences than those who received a placebo.

Side Effects: Nausea, flushing, and headache are frequent side effects. Additionally, it may result in a rise in blood pressure, which needs to be watched.

Treatment with testosterone replacement:

Both men and women need testosterone, and low testosterone levels can cause women to have less of a desire for sex. It's possible that testosterone replacement therapy will help some women with HSDD.

Modalities of action: the goals of testosterone replacement therapy to replenish low testosterone levels in female patients.

Testosterone therapy can be given in a number of different ways, such as patches, gels, and injections. The right dosage and form depend on the needs and preferences of the individual.

Effectiveness: In women with established testosterone deficiency, testosterone replacement therapy can increase sexual desire. It is not advised for all women with HSDD, and a healthcare professional should closely monitor its use.

Possible side effects of testosterone therapy for women include voice deepening, hair growth, and acne. Higher doses are more likely to cause these side effects.

4. HRT: Hormone Replacement Therapy

The main purpose of hormone replacement therapy, which contains oestrogen and/or progesterone, is to treat menopausal symptoms. Possibly indirectly increase the desire for sex in menopausal-related HSDD women.

HRT works by balancing a woman's hormone levels whether she is menopausal or postmenopausal.

Dosage and Administration: Individual needs and symptom patterns determine the dosage and regimen of HRT.

Effectiveness: HRT can reduce menopausal symptoms like vaginal dryness and discomfort, which can help some women feel more sexually attracted to and satisfied with themselves.

HRT frequently causes bloating, mood swings, and breast tenderness as side effects. The choice to use HRT should be carefully considered in consultation with a healthcare professional because there are potential risks linked to long-term HRT, such as an increased risk of cardiovascular events and breast cancer.

5. Psychological Therapy and Counselling:

Low sexual desire is a frequent problem in Psychological issues in women, such as stress, anxiety, depression, or relationship problems, may be to blame. In order to address these underlying causes, psychotherapy or counselling can be very effective.

Mechanism of Action: Therapy offers women a safe space to explore and comprehend the psychological and emotional factors influencing their low sex drive. Additionally, it can enhance communication skills and teach coping mechanisms.

Effectiveness: In many cases of HSDD, therapy has been shown to be helpful, especially when psychological or interpersonal problems are the root causes.

Side Effects: Psychotherapy and counselling typically have no negative side effects. It is regarded as a reliable and advantageous option for treating HSDD.

6. Changes in Lifestyle:

Stress, a poor diet, inactivity, and fatigue are all examples of lifestyle factors that can sexual desire in a negative way. Making improvements in these areas can have a big impact on libido.

Mechanism of Action: Changing your lifestyle can improve your overall health, lower your stress level, and give you more energy, all of which have a positive impact on your desire for sex.

Dosage and administration: Making lifestyle changes calls for ongoing dedication and work. A balanced diet, regular exercise, stress-reduction methods, and enough sleep are a few examples.

Effectiveness: For some women, modifying their lifestyles can significantly increase their sexual desire and sexual satisfaction.

Generally speaking, leading a healthy lifestyle has no negative side effects.

7. Developing Relationships and Communication : Communication with a partner in an open and honest manner can be beneficial when relationship problems or communication issues cause lack of sexual desire strategy.

Improved communication and emotional closeness can aid in addressing relationship-related issues that might be adversely affecting sexual desire.

Effectiveness: Increasing sexual satisfaction and desire can be attained by fortifying the emotional bond and resolving relationship problems.

Improvements in communication and relationship building typically have no negative side effects.

Conclusion:

Low sex desire in women, or HSDD, is a problem that affects a lot of women and can be very detrimental to their general health and quality of life. Flibanserin (Addyi), bremelanotide (Vyleesi), testosterone replacement therapy, hormone replacement therapy (HRT), psychological counselling, dietary changes, and relationship and communication improvement techniques are just a few of the medications and treatment modalities that are available to address this condition.

It's critical for women who lack sexual desire to speak with a physician. in order to identify the root causes of their condition and investigate the best available treatments. Individual treatment plans should be chosen after taking into account the underlying causes of HSDD, potential side effects, and patient preferences. In order to address and resolve problems associated with low sexual desire in women, open and honest communication with a healthcare professional and, when appropriate, with a partner, is crucial.

OSPHENA

Osphena is a drug that was created to treat a specific issue in postmenopausal women called dyspareunia, which is marked by uncomfortable sex. It's important to remember that Osphena is a drug intended to reduce pain during sexual activity rather than to boost sexual desire (libido).

Mechanism of Action: Ospemifene, a selective oestrogen receptor modulator (SERM), is the active component of Osphena. It functions by attaching to oestrogen receptors in the vaginal tissue, increasing the elasticity and lubrication of the vagina. This may lessen the discomfort of sexual activity for postmenopausal women.

Osphena has been given FDA approval to treat postmenopausal women with moderate to severe dyspareunia (painful intercourse) brought on by vulvovaginal atrophy (VVA). A condition known as VVA is characterised by a Vaginal wall thinning and inflammation can be brought on by menopause's decreased oestrogen levels.

Dosage and Administration: One 60 mg tablet taken orally once daily with food is the usual dosage for Osphena. For their particular symptoms, women should use the lowest effective dose, and treatment should be reviewed on a regular basis.

Effectiveness: According to clinical studies, Osphena effectively reduces the dyspareunia symptoms experienced by postmenopausal women by enhancing vaginal lubrication and minimising vaginal dryness. Osphena does not treat other menopause symptoms like hot flashes or night sweats, which must be kept in mind.

Potential Side Effects: Osphena frequently causes hot flashes, vaginal discharge, muscle spasms, and perspiration. A few women might have an increased risk of endometrial cancer, blood clots, and stroke. Osphena is therefore typically advised for women who cannot or do not want to use estrogen-based therapies for VVA.

Precautions and considerations: Women thinking about taking

Osphena should talk to their doctor about their medical history and any possible risk factors. People with a history of breast cancer, heart disease, liver issues, or blood clots should pay particular attention to this.

Osphena is a drug that has been approved for postmenopausal women who experience painful sex because of vulvovaginal atrophy. It functions by enhancing the elasticity and lubrication of the vagina. Although it can be a useful treatment for dyspareunia, it's crucial for women to discuss the advantages, potential risks, and alternatives with their healthcare provider to ascertain if it's right for them.

Osphena is the ideal course of treatment for their particular requirements and situation.

The FDA granted Addyi, also referred to by its generic name flibanserin, approval in 2015 to treat premenopausal women with hypoactive sexual desire disorder (HSDD). A persistent and distressing lack of sexual desire or interest, which results in emotional distress and lowers a woman's quality of life overall, is the hallmark of HSDD.

Addyi functions differently from drugs like Viagra that are intended to treat male sexual dysfunction. It is both a serotonin 1A receptor agonist and an antagonist of the serotonin 2A receptor. This indicates that it primarily affects brain neurotransmitters, concentrating on serotonin and dopamine levels. Addyi aims to increase sexual desire and enhance overall sexual satisfaction by rebalancing these neurotransmitters.

Use and Indications: Addyi is recommended for the treatment of HSDD in premenopausal women is acquired and generalised. It's important to remember that Addyi is not meant to be used by postmenopausal people, either men or women.

Administration and Dosage: The suggested dosage for Addyi is one 100 mg tablet taken orally once daily before bed. It should be taken with food because taking it on an empty stomach may make side effects more likely. If a woman's sexual desire does not improve after eight weeks of treatment, she should be advised to stop.

Effectiveness: Based on clinical trials, women taking Addyi had a marginally higher sex desire than women taking a placebo. It's crucial to note that the improvement is only considered to be moderate, and Addyi may not be successful for all sufferers of HSDD. Furthermore, different women may react differently to Addyi, and it might take some time before sexual desire improves.

Potential Side Effects: Addyi frequently causes side effects such as drowsiness, somnolence, nausea, fatigue, and dry mouth. It is advised that women refrain from engaging in tasks requiring mental clarity, such as operating a motor vehicle, until they are familiar with how Addyi affects them because these side effects can be severe.

Addyi carries the FDA's most severe type of warning, known as a "Boxed Warning," along with a list of contraindications. The risk of severe hypotension (low blood pressure) and syncope (fainting) when taking Addyi is highlighted in this warning, particularly when it is combined with alcohol, certain prescription drugs, or in patients with liver disease impairment.

The following circumstances are contraindicated for using Addyi:

Alcohol use concurrently due to the possibility of syncope and severe hypotension.

patients who have previously experienced Addyi hypersensitivity reactions.

Patients with hepatic impairment because of the possibility of negative drug effects and increased drug exposure.

Addyi is a drug that has been approved to treat HSDD in

premenopausal women, which deals with a lack of sexual desire that causes emotional distress. It differs from drugs like Viagra and increases sexual desire by affecting the brain's neurotransmitters.

Addyi comes with important caveats, such as the possibility of side effects and interactions with alcohol and specific medications, even though it may be effective for some women. Women with HSDD should speak with their healthcare provider in-depth about Analyse the potential advantages and disadvantages and decide whether Addyi is a suitable treatment option for their particular situation. To address sexual health issues safely and effectively, it is crucial to consult a healthcare professional.

Title: Vyleesi (Bremelanotide): A Comprehensive Guide to Libido Enhancement in Women

INTRODUCTION

Bremelanotide, the brand name of the drug known as

Vyleesi, is used to treat Hypoactive Sexual Desire Disorder (HSDD), a specific and frequently disregarded issue affecting women's sexual health. A woman's quality of life and her intimate relationships can be significantly impacted by HSDD, which is characterised by a distressing and persistent lack of sexual interest or desire. Women looking to regain their sexual desire and fulfilment may find a potential solution in Vyleesi, which represents a fresh and cutting-edge approach to treating this condition.

HSDD comprehension

It's important to understand the significance of HSDD and how it impacts women's lives before delving into Vyleesi's mechanism of action and application. HSDD is a condition with many different manifestations that can be caused by a number of elements, such as psychological, emotional, and physiological ones. Here are some crucial HSDD features:

Prevalence: HSDD is a problem that affects women of all ages and is relatively common. It can strike both premenopausal and postmenopausal women, and as women get older, it becomes more common.

HSDD is frequently associated with psychological conditions like stress, anxiety, depression, low self-esteem, or past trauma. These emotional factors may hinder sexual arousal and desire.

Relationship Dynamics: HSDD can be exacerbated by relationship issues like poor communication, unresolved conflicts, or a lack of emotional intimacy. For a fulfilling sexual life, a healthy relationship and open communication are essential.

Physical Health: A number of medical conditions, including chronic illnesses, hormonal imbalances, and diabetes, can to reduce sexual lust. The libido may be impacted by the medications used to treat these conditions.

Hormonal Changes: Hormone swings, particularly during menopause, can alter one's desire for sexual activity. Sexual activity may seem less appealing due to dryness and discomfort in the vaginal area caused by a drop in oestrogen levels.

Cultural and societal factors can affect a woman's perception of her own desires and her willingness to speak about or seek help for HSDD. These factors include cultural or societal norms, religious beliefs, and societal stigmas surrounding sexuality.

Enter Vyleesi: A Novel HSDD Approach

The FDA has approved Vyleesi, also referred to by its generic name bremelanotide, as a treatment for acquired, generalised HSDD in premenopausal women. In contrast to earlier therapies for HSDD, which primarily focused on hormonal or psychological factors, Vyleesi acts on the central nervous system to boost desire for sexual activity.

Process of action

The mechanism of action of Vyleesi sets it apart from other HSDD treatments. It specifically targets the brain's melanocortin receptors as a melanocortin receptor agonist. Sexual response and desire are greatly influenced by these receptors.

The melanocortin receptors are activated when a woman takes Vyleesi, which increases her desire and interest for sex. This action takes place at the neural level and addresses how the brain controls sexual desire.

ADMINISTRATION AND USE

At least 45 minutes before the planned sexual activity,

Vyleesi is administered as a self-injection into the thigh or abdomen. Women now have the freedom to take the medication as needed, encouraging the spontaneity of sex.

It is It's important to remember that women shouldn't take Vyleesi more than eight times per month and shouldn't take it more than once every 24 hours. For it to work best and to have the fewest side effects possible, use it responsibly and in accordance with the suggested dosing instructions.

EFFECTIVENESS

Women who took bremelanotide (Vyleesi) reported slightly more sexual desire and more satisfying sexual experiences than those who took a placebo, according to clinical trials. Even though the improvement is regarded as moderate, Vyleesi offers HSDD sufferers an important alternative, particularly when other methods of treatment have failed.

It's important to remember that everyone's reaction to Vyleesi will be different. Some women might encounter a more significant improvement in sexual desire and satisfaction, while others may have a milder response. As with many medications, the effectiveness of Vyleesi may depend on individual factors, including the underlying causes of HSDD.

SIDE EFFECTS AND SAFETY

Like all medications, Vyleesi comes with potential side effects. It's essential to be aware of these side effects and discuss them with a healthcare provider before using the medication. Common side effects of Vyleesi may include:

Nausea: Some women may experience mild to moderate nausea after taking Vyleesi. Taking the medication with food can help reduce this side effect.

Flushing: Flushing, characterized by redness and warmth in the face and upper body, can occur after Vyleesi administration. This side effect is generally temporary and mild. significant improvement in sexual desire and satisfaction, while others may have a milder response. As with many medications, the effectiveness of Vyleesi may depend on individual factors, including the underlying causes of HSDD.

SIDE EFFECTS AND SAFETY

Like all medications, Vyleesi comes with potential side effects. It's essential to be aware of these side effects and discuss them with a healthcare provider before using the medication. Common side effects of Vyleesi may include:

Nausea: Some women may experience mild to moderate nausea after taking Vyleesi. Taking the medication with food can help reduce this side effect.

Flushing: Flushing, characterized by redness and warmth in the face and upper body, can occur after Vyleesi administration. This side effect is generally temporary and mild.

Headache: Headaches are another potential side effect of Vyleesi. They are typically mild to moderate in intensity.

Injection Site Reactions: Women may experience discomfort or minor irritation at the injection site. Proper technique and site rotation can minimize this side effect.

It's important to consult with a healthcare provider to determine if Vyleesi is a suitable option and to discuss strategies for managing potential side effects. It's worth noting that Vyleesi has been well-tolerated in clinical trials, and the majority of side effects reported were mild to moderate in severity.

Safety Considerations

Before considering Vyleesi, women should discuss their medical history and any potential risk factors with their healthcare provider. It's important to inform the healthcare provider about any medications, supplements, or health conditions, especially if they may interact with Vyleesi or affect its safety and efficacy.

Women with certain medical conditions, such as uncontrolled hypertension (high blood pressure), cardiovascular disease, or a history of melanoma, may not be suitable candidates for Vyleesi. Additionally, Vyleesi's safety during pregnancy or breastfeeding has not been established, so it should not be used in these situations.

Conclusion

Vyleesi (bremelanotide) represents a significant advancement in the treatment of Hypoactive Sexual Desire Disorder (HSDD) in premenopausal women. This medication offers a novel approach to addressing HSDD by acting on the central nervous system to increase sexual desire.

While Vyleesi has demonstrated effectiveness in clinical trials, it's essential to recognize that individual responses may vary. It provides women with a valuable option for managing HSDD, especially when other treatments or approaches have not been effective.

Women considering Vyleesi should have open and honest discussions with their healthcare providers to assess its suitability for their specific needs and circumstances. By understanding the medication's mechanism of action, proper use, potential side effects, and safety considerations, women can make informed decisions about incorporating Vyleesi into their approach to addressing HSDD and enhancing their overall sexual well-being.

a notable increase in sexual desire and satisfaction, whereas some people may experience a milder response. The effectiveness of Vyleesi may vary from person to person and may be influenced by a variety of variables, including the underlying causes of HSDD.

Safety and negative effects

Vyleesi may cause side effects, just like all medications. Before taking the medication, you must be aware of these side effects and talk to your doctor about them. Vyleesi's typical side effects may include:

After taking Vyleesi, some women may experience mild to moderate nausea. This side effect can be lessened by taking the medication with food.

Flushing: Flushing, characterised by warmth and redness in the upper body and face, can happen after taking Vyleesi. Typically, this adverse effect is brief and minor.

Migraine: Migraines are Vyleesi might also have a negative side effect. Usually, they range from mild to moderate in intensity.

Reactions at the Injection Site: Women may feel a little achy or irritated at the Injection Site. This side effect can be reduced with appropriate technique and site rotation.

It's crucial to speak with a healthcare professional to decide whether Vyleesi is a good option and to go over management options for any potential side effects. It's important to note that

Vyleesi has a good safety profile, with the majority of side effects reported being mild to moderate in severity.

Considerations for Safety

Women should speak with their healthcare provider about their medical history and any potential risk factors before considering Vyleesi. Any medications, dietary supplements, or medical conditions must be disclosed to the healthcare provider, especially if they mays interact with Vyleesi or compromise its effectiveness and safety.

Vyleesi may not be appropriate for women with certain medical conditions, such as uncontrolled hypertension (high blood pressure), cardiovascular disease, or a history of melanoma. Vyleesi shouldn't be used in these circumstances because it hasn't been proven to be safe during pregnancy or breast-feeding.

Conclusion

The medication Vyleesi (bremelanotide) represents a significant improvement in the way premenopausal women with Hypoactive Sexual Desire Disorder (HSDD) are treated. By stimulating sexual desire by acting on the central nervous system, this medication offers a novel method for treating HSDD.

Although Vyleesi has shown effectiveness in clinical trials, it's important to understand that different people may respond differently. In particular when other treatments are ineffective, it gives women a beneficial alternative for managing HSDD our strategies have not worked.

In order to determine whether Vyleesi is a good fit for their particular needs and circumstances, women who are considering it should have open and honest discussions with their healthcare professionals. Women can decide whether to include Vyleesi in their strategy for treating HSDD and improving their general sexual well-being by being aware of the medication's mechanism of action, proper use, potential side effects, and safety considerations.

CHAPTER THREE

Dosages, Mechanism of Action and Side Effects of female Viagra

Introduction

Female Viagra, also known as flibanserin, has drawn a lot of interest as a possible cure for female sexual dysfunction (FSD). FSD includes a number of conditions that cause significant distress in women and are characterised by a persistent lack of sexual desire and arousal. In contrast to the sildenafil-focused Viagra (for men), this medication caters to the specific needs of female patients with erectile dysfunction. To give readers a complete understanding of the use, effectiveness, and potential risks of female Viagra, this in-depth review will examine the dosages, mechanism of action, and side effects of the drug.

I. Female Viagra (Flibanserin) dosage Different dosages of flibanserin, also known as Female Viagra, are offered to accommodate individual needs and reduce any potential side effects. The drug can primarily be found in It is consumed orally in tablet form.

suggested dosage

100 mg once daily at bedtime is the starting dose for female Viagra (flibanserin). Healthcare professionals must stress the importance of taking the medication at bedtime to lower the risk of side effects like low blood pressure and dizziness, which can become worse when taken during the day. The purpose of taking the medication at bedtime is to allow the medication to work while the patient is sleeping, potentially reducing these side effects.

Dose Modification

Healthcare professionals must keep track of the patient's response to the initial dosage and modify it as necessary. If the 100 mg first dose is not well tolerated or does not sufficiently improve arousal and sexual desire, a higher dose of 200 mg should be tried. 100 mg once daily is the maximum dose that can be gradually increased.

Treatment Time Frame

Individuals may respond to flibanserin for a different amount of time. For an evaluation of the treatment's efficacy, it is advised to continue it for at least 8 weeks. Patients and medical professionals influences the chemistry of the brain.

Changes in Serotonin Receptors

A specific serotonin receptor modulator is flobanserin. It functions by attaching to serotonin receptors, specifically the 5-HT1A receptor subtype, and decreasing serotonin activity in the prefrontal cortex of the brain at the same time. This dual action restores the serotonin-dopamine ratio, which is essential for controlling arousal and sexual desire.

Higher Dopamine and Norepinephrine levels

Flibanserin increases the release of dopamine and norepinephrine, two neurotransmitters linked to increased sexual interest and responsiveness, by decreasing serotonin activity. Some women taking the medication report an improvement in their sexual desire as a result of this alteration in neurotransmitter balance.

Advanced Mechanism

Flibanserin's mechanism of action is intricate and poorly

understood. It requires a careful balance between should consult frequently to decide on the right course of treatment, taking into account each patient's needs and medication response.

2. Action Mechanism

Understanding how female Viagra (flibanserin) affects female sexual desire and arousal requires knowledge of the drug's mechanism of action.

Dopamine and Serotonin

Flibanserin targets particular neurotransmitters, primarily serotonin and dopamine, acting on the central nervous system. Flibanserin functions differently from sildenafil, which primarily increases blood flow to the genital region. Individuals may respond differently to different neurotransmitters and their effects. As more is learned about the precise mechanisms, it will become clearer how effective it might be in treating FSD.

3. Female Viagra (Flibanserin) Side Effects

Female Viagra (flibanserin) is linked to a variety of potential side effects, just like any medication. For patients and healthcare professionals to choose appropriate treatments, they must be aware of these side effects.

Typical Adverse Effects

The most typical flibanserin side effects include:

Dizziness

Fatigue

Nausea

Mouth ache

These negative effects are frequently minor and usually go away with continued use. To ascertain whether dosage adjustments or alternative treatments are required, patients must discuss any bothersome side effects with their healthcare provider.

Low Blood Pressure Taking flibanserin during the day, in particular, can lower blood pressure. Symptoms like dizziness, lightheadedness, and fainting may result from this. The medication is typically taken before bed to reduce this risk. Alcohol shouldn't be consumed by patients who are taking flibanserin because it can make their low blood pressure worse.

Relationship to Alcohol

The interaction of flibanserin with alcohol is a significant area of concern. When taking the medication, drinking alcohol can significantly increase the risk of severe hypotension and syncope. Patients taking flibanserin should be strongly advised by their medical professionals to avoid drinking alcohol.

Effects on the Central Nervous System

While taking flibanserin, some patients may experience effects on the central nervous system like drowsiness and somnolence. These effects may make it more difficult for someone to perform attention-demanding tasks, like driving. Patients should be advised to avoid alertnessdemanding activities until they understand how the medication affects them.

Assessment of Hypoactive Sexual Desire Disorder (HSDD)

Healthcare professionals should examine patients for Hypoactive Sexual Desire Disorder (HSDD) before prescribing flibanserin. For premenopausal women with HSDD, which is characterised by a persistent lack of sexual desire that causes personal distress, the medication is specifically advised.

Personal Reaction

It's crucial to remember that every person will react to flibanserin differently. While some women may notice significant improvements in arousal and sexual desire with few side effects, others may not find the medication to be effective or may experience negative side effects that outweigh the positive effects.

Speaking with a healthcare professional

Patients need to be given a Before beginning treatment, patients should have a thorough discussion with their doctor about the potential advantages and disadvantages of flibanserin. Making decisions about the suitability of this medication for a specific person's circumstances requires open communication.

CONCLUSION

Flibanserin, also known as female Viagra, is an option for treating premenopausal women with Hypoactive Sexual Desire Disorder (HSDD). Important factors to take into account for patients and healthcare professionals alike include its dosages, mode of action, and side effects.

Flibanserin is typically prescribed in doses that begin at 100 mg once daily at bedtime, with a maximum dose adjustment of 100 mg. Each patient's course of treatment is unique, and the length should be decided in consultation with a medical professional.

Flibanserin's mechanism of action entails the alteration of serotonin and dopamine levels in the brain, which could possibly increase arousal and sexual desire

While flibanserin may be helpful for some women, it is also frequently connected to unpleasant side effects like fatigue, nausea, dry mouth, and dizziness. Additionally, it may cause central nervous system side effects like sleepiness and lower blood pressure, particularly when combined with alcohol. To properly assess potential benefits versus risks and to effectively monitor and manage side effects, patients should have a thorough conversation with their healthcare provider.

In conclusion, flibanserin is a medication that specifically targets a problem with women's sexual health and calls for careful consideration from both healthcare professionals and patients to ensure its safe and efficient use. as continuing study advances our understanding of FSD and its treatment options, it is essential to stay informed about the latest developments in this field

THE EFFECTIVINESS OF FLIBANSERIN

Treatment of Hypoactive Sexual Desire Disorder (HSDD) with Flibanserin

Abstract:

Millions of women worldwide suffer from the common and distressing condition known as Hypoactive Sexual Desire Disorder (HSDD). An FDA-approved drug called libanserin was developed to deal with this problem. The efficacy of flibanserin in the management of HSDD is examined in this extensive review. We investigate its mode of action, clinical studies, adverse effects, and function in relation to other HSDD treatment options.

INTRODUCTION

A complex sexual dysfunction known as hypoactive sexual desire disorder (HSDD) is characterised by a persistent lack of sexual desire, which can be distressing for people and frequently put strain on relationships. According to estimates, HSDD could have an impact on up to 10% of women. The focus of this review is the efficiency of flibanserin in treating HSDD, a a long-standing underdiagnosed and under-treated condition.

Mechanism of Action of Flibanserin: The U.S. Food and Drug Administration (FDA) approved the drug flibanserin in 2015 for the treatment of HSDD in premenopausal women. It is sold under the trade name Addyi. The medication affects the central nervous system by specifically acting on the dopamine and serotonin receptors. Flibanserin aims to address the complex psychological factors associated with HSDD, in contrast to many other medications for sexual dysfunction that primarily focus on blood flow.

Clinical Trial Efficacy: To assess flibanserin's effectiveness in treating HSDD, several clinical trials have been carried out. We go over the planning, outcomes, and implications of these studies to shed light on the drug's efficiency in enhancing female sexual desire and elevating overall sexual satisfaction in women.

Safety profile and side effects:

Like any medication, libbanserin has side effects. We offer a thorough breakdown of the possible negative effects, their frequency, and the implications for patients. To assist medical professionals and patients in making wise choices regarding the use of flibanserin, the risk-benefit ratio of the drug is discussed.

COMPARATIVE EVALUATION OF OTHER TREATMENT POSSIBILITIES:

A number of therapeutic approaches, such as lifestyle modifications, psychological counselling, and complementary medications, can be used to manage HSDD. This review investigates how flibanserin compares to these complementary therapies and determines whether it is an appropriate option for various patient populations.

CLINICAL PRACTISE IN THE REAL WORLD:

In addition to clinical trials, actual clinical experience and patient reviews offer important insights into the efficacy of flibanserin. We use actual data to provide a more comprehensive analysis.

Why Menopausal Women Are More Susceptible To

This HSDD (Hypoactive Sexual Desire Disorder)

Due to a confluence of hormonal, psychological, and physiological changes that take place both during and after menopause, menopausal women are more prone to developing Hypoactive Sexual Desire Disorder (HSDD). The hallmark of HSDD is a persistent lack of sexual desire, which can be extremely distressing and have a detrimental effect on a person's quality of life. Let's examine the factors that contribute to menopausal women having a higher risk of HSDD:

1. Hormonal Modifications

The production of sex hormones, particularly oestrogen and progesterone, as well as testosterone on occasion, significantly declines during menopause. In controlling sexual arousal and desire, these hormones are extremely important. Women's libidos may decline as their levels drop throughout and after menopause, making them more susceptible to HSDD. particularly testosterone.

Is Taking Viagra Everyday Good For You?

Unless specifically advised by a healthcare professional for a particular medical condition, taking Viagra (sildenafil) daily is not advised. The primary purpose of Viagra is to treat erectile dysfunction (ED), a condition marked by the inability to obtain or maintain an erection strong enough for sexual activity. Here are some crucial factors to remember:

Viagra is a prescription drug that needs to be taken under the direction and supervision of a trained healthcare professional. Use of it without a prescription is not advised.

Viagra is used to treat erectile dysfunction and is typically taken between 30 minutes and 4 hours before sexual activity. It is not intended to be taken every day by people without ED.

Like any medication, Viagra may cause side effects side effects, which can occasionally be more serious, can include headache, facial flushing, upset stomach, and others. It's possible that taking it frequently will make these side effects more likely to occur.

Daily use of Viagra can cause tolerance, which results in the drug losing some of its effectiveness over time. Higher doses might be necessary, which raises the possibility of negative side effects.

Viagra can affect blood pressure, and it can be dangerous for people who already have certain preexisting medical conditions, like cardiovascular problems. It might be risky to use it frequently without the proper medical supervision.

Drug Interaction: Viagra can interact with other medicines and have adverse effects that could be harmful. A healthcare professional can evaluate possible drug interactions and modify treatment as necessary.

Psychological Dependence: Using Viagra consistently over an extended period of time has the potential to cause psychological dependence, in which the user begins to feel they are sexually ineffective without the drug. It is crucial to speak with a healthcare provider if you have sexual health issues or are experiencing erectile dysfunction. They are able to assess your particular situation, identify the underlying causes of your condition, and suggest suitable treatment options, which could entail making lifestyle changes, going through psychotherapy, or taking medications like Viagra if it is determined that they are appropriate in your situation. Viagra self-medication is not advised because it may result in health risks and may not address the underlying causes of your sexual health issues. For the best and safest course of treatment, always seek advice from a medical professional.

HOW TO OBTAIN VIAGRA

You should adhere to a safe and legal procedure in order to

obtain Viagra (sildenafil), a prescription drug for the treatment of erectile dysfunction (ED). The following is a general how-to for obtaining Viagra:

CONSULT A MEDICAL PROFESSIONAL

The initial and most important step is to speak with a healthcare professional. You should schedule a consultation with a physician, urologist, or other healthcare provider who can examine your medical history, present symptoms, and general state of health. If Viagra is a suitable treatment for your particular circumstance, they will decide that.

MEDICAL ASSESSMENT

Your healthcare provider will perform a thorough medical evaluation during the consultation, which may include talking about your medical history, lifestyle choices, and the severity of your ED. Be truthful and upfront about any existing medical issues or medications you are taking and your general well-being.

AN EXAMINATION OF THE BODY

A physical examination might be necessary, depending on your healthcare provider's evaluation. While not always required, it can aid in locating any underlying physical causes of ED.

Discussion of Potential Therapies: In addition to discussing treatment options with you, your doctor will go over Viagra's mechanism of action. They will also talk about the risks and potential side effects of Viagra. You might also look into complementary therapies and way of life adjustments that can enhance your sexual health.

An order for Viagra: If your doctor decides Viagra is a good option for treating your erectile dysfunction, they will write a prescription. This prescription details the medication, the dosage, and the recommended dosage. Throughout this consultation, you should address any uncertainties you may have about using Viagra.

Decide on a pharmacy: You can select a pharmacy to fill your Viagra prescription once you have one. You can choose between an online pharmacy and a neighbourhood brick-and-mortar pharmacy, but make sure the pharmacy is reputable and licenced.

Drugstore Consultation: You might occasionally have an additional consultation with a healthcare professional connected to the online pharmacy when using one. To determine whether it is appropriate to dispense you with Viagra, they will review your prescription and your medical history.

BUYING VIAGRA

The chosen pharmacy will let you buy Viagra after consultation and approval. Make sure to give them the prescription so they can give you the medicine as directed.

Reviewing the prescription instructions:

It is crucial to read and comprehend the directions for using the medication Seek immediate medical attention if you have an extended or painful erection (priapism) that lasts longer than four hours as this can be a serious side effect.

Potential Alternatives to the Medicine Viagra

For the treatment of erectile dysfunction (ED), Viagra (sildenafil) has a number of potential substitutes. The individual's health, preferences, and the underlying causes of ED all factor into the treatment decision. Here are a few typical substitutes: Drugs taken orally:

a. Tadalafil (Cialis): A PDE-5 inhibitor similar to Viagra, Cialis is taken as needed. It has a longer duration of action and is frequently referred to as a "weekend pill" because of how long its effects can last.

b.   Vardenafil, also known as Levitra, is a PDE-5 inhibitor that functions similarly to Viagra. For those who do not respond well to Viagra, it might be an alternative.

Medicines taken externally:

Alprostadil (Caverject, Edex, MUSE) is a medication that comes in a variety of forms, such as injections, suppositories, and urethral sprays. It is used to dilate blood vessels and improve blood flow to the penis. Alprostadil is often used when oral medications are ineffective or not well-tolerated.

b. Avanafil (Stendra): Avanafil is another PDE-5 inhibitor similar to Viagra, known for its fast onset of action, often within 15 minutes. Lifestyle Changes:

a. Diet and Exercise: Improving cardiovascular health through a healthy diet and regular exercise can enhance blood flow, which is vital for erectile function.

b. Smoking Cessation: Quitting smoking can improve blood flow and overall health, potentially alleviating ED.

c. Weight Management: Maintaining a healthy weight can reduce the risk of ED, as obesity is a risk factor.

d. Alcohol and Substance Abuse Reduction: Reducing or eliminating alcohol and drug use can improve sexual function.

Psychological Counseling:

ED can often have psychological causes. Counseling, either alone or in conjunction with other treatments, may help address issues like anxiety, depression, or performance-related stress.

Vacuum Erection Devices (VEDs):

A VED is a non-invasive device that creates a vacuum around the penis, drawing blood into it to produce an erection. A constriction ring is then placed at the base to maintain the erection.

Penile Implants:

Penile implants are surgically inserted devices that can provide an erection when desired. They are considered when other treatments have failed or are not well-tolerated.

VYLEESI

Testosterone Replacement Therapy:

In cases where ED is related to low testosterone levels (hypogonadism), testosterone replacement therapy may be considered.

Herbal Supplements:

Some individuals explore herbal remedies like ginseng, Larginine, or yohimbine. However, the efficacy and safety of these supplements are often not well-established, and they should be used with caution.

Shockwave Therapy:

Low-intensity shockwave therapy (LI-ESWT) is a relatively new treatment for ED. It involves using acoustic waves to stimulate the growth of new blood vessels in the penis, potentially improving blood flow.

Pelvic Floor Exercises:

Pelvic floor exercises, such as Kegel exercises, may be recommended as part of a broader treatment plan for ED.

It is essential to consult with a healthcare provider before pursuing any alternative treatment for ED. They can help determine the underlying causes of your condition and guide you toward the most appropriate treatment options. ED can result from various factors, including medical conditions, medications, lifestyle, and psychological factors. Therefore, an accurate diagnosis is crucial for effective treatment. Remember that while many alternatives to Viagra are available, the best choice depends on your specific needs and the recommendations of your healthcare provider

Not everyone is a candidate for Viagra. Viagra should not be taken by men with certain medical conditions, such as severe heart issues, recent strokes, or use of nitrate medications. Your medical professional will determine your eligibility.

Any worries, queries, or side effects you may encounter while taking Viagra must be discussed honestly and openly with your doctor.

Alternative treatments, such as other prescription drugs or medical procedures, may be taken into consideration if Viagra is ineffective or has unpleasant side effects.

In order to ensure that Viagra is used safely and effectively, the process of obtaining it is regulated. Always seek advice from a doctor to talk about your unique needs and, if necessary for your condition, get a prescription.

The drug Viagra (sildenafil) helps men achieve and maintain erections by improving blood flow to the penis. It is typically prescribed to treat erectile dysfunction (ED). The length of Viagra's effects varies from person to person and is influenced by a number of variables. What you need to know about how long Viagra's effects last is as follows:

Action Begins:

After ingestion, Viagra typically begins to work 30 to 60 minutes later. However, depending on your personal metabolism, what you've eaten, and your general health, the onset can change.

Continuity of Effect:

In most cases, Viagra's effects last for four to six hours. During this time, a man's ability to get and keep an erection when sexually aroused improves. This is not to say that an ongoing erection during this time doesn't necessarily mean that the response to sexual stimulation is getting better.

Time and Food:

When taking Viagra with a large, high-fat meal, its onset of action may be delayed. For quickest results, it is typically advised to take Viagra on an empty stomach. Furthermore, the timing of sexual activity can affect Viagra's efficiency. Planning sexual activity within the 4 to 6 hour window of its anticipated effect is essential.

Individual Response and Dose:

Depending on the dose, the effects of Viagra may last a shorter or longer time. There are three different strengths of Viagra: 25 mg, 50 mg, and 100 mg. Higher doses might last longer, but they also come with a higher chance of side effects.

Individual Differences: Individuals may experience Viagra's effects for a different amount of time. While some men may only experience the medication's effects for the first four hours, others may feel its effects for much longer. Additional Doses:

It is generally not advised to take a second dose of Viagra within 24 hours unless directed to do so by a healthcare professional. Doubling the dose increases the risk of side effects rather than necessarily extending the duration of the effects.

Adaptation and Tolerance:

Due to the emergence of tolerance, some men may notice a reduction in the duration of Viagra's effectiveness over time. At this point, the body stops responding as well to the medication. If this happens, a healthcare professional might suggest different therapies or dosing regimens.

Aspects of Safety Effects:

While Viagra is generally considered safe when taken as directed, it is essential to be aware of potential side effects and discontinue use if you experience severe or intolerable side effects.

Longer-Lasting Alternatives:If a longer duration of effect is desired, there are alternative medications available. For example, tadalafil (Cialis) has a longer duration of action, with effects lasting up to 36 hours. This has earned it the nickname "the weekend pill."

Consult a Healthcare Provider:

It is crucial to consult a healthcare provider before using Viagra or any other ED medication. They can help determine the most suitable treatment based on your individual needs and health conditions.

In summary, Viagra typically starts working within 30 minutes to an hour and has an effective duration of about 4 to 6 hours. The duration can vary between individuals and may be influenced by factors like dose, food, and individual response. Always follow your healthcare provider's guidance regarding the appropriate use of Viagra to maximize its benefits and minimize the risk of side effects.

Who would stand a gain from this?

Viagra is a well-known medication that is typically prescribed for the treatment of erectile dysfunction (ED), which is of interest to a wide range of stakeholders. These parties involved include:

Pharmaceutical Firms: Pfizer is one pharmaceutical firm that has a sizable interest in Viagra. They are the owners of the patents and the commercial rights to produce, market, and sell the medication, making it a profitable good.

Healthcare Professionals: Since they recommend Viagra to patients with ED, healthcare professionals like doctors, urologists, and other specialists have an interest in the drug. They are in charge of determining whether patients are suitable for the medication, going over how to use it, and keeping an eye on its results.

Patients: Men with ED are particularly interested in Viagra because it may help them treat their condition. It can significantly enhance their general well-being, relationships, and quality of life well-being.

Pharmacists: Pharmacists are in charge of providing patients with a valid prescription with Viagra. Additionally, they give advice and information on how to use it properly and any possible drug interactions.

Health Insurance Companies: When it comes to coverage and reimbursement guidelines, health insurance companies are interested in Viagra. ED medication costs are covered by some insurance plans, but others might ask patients to pay out-of-pocket. Researchers and Scientists: Researchers are interested in learning more about how Viagra works and how it affects people in order to explore potential applications for the drug beyond ED.

Regulatory Organisations: In the United States, regulatory organisations like the Food and Drug Administration (FDA) are very interested in ensuring the efficacy, safety, and accurate labelling of medicines like Viagra. They sanction and control how it is used on the market.

Public health organisations: The World Health Organisation (WHO) and local health departments, as well as other organisations with a focus on sexual and reproductive health, have an interest in promoting the responsible and safe use of ED drugs like Viagra.

Marketing and advertising firms: These businesses have an interest in promoting Viagra to patients and healthcare professionals. This includes launching campaigns for education and awareness.

Legal and Ethical Watchdogs: Organisations and people concerned with the legal and ethical aspects of pharmaceutical marketing and distribution keep an eye on Viagra's promotion and advertising strategies to make sure they abide by the law and moral principles.

Advocacy Groups: ED and other sexual health issues are the focus of advocacy groups. They strive to promote access to ED treatments, which may include Viagra, by increasing awareness, offering support, and speaking out.

Producers of Generic Versions: Businesses that make generic versions of sildenafil, the substance that powers Viagra, have a stake in this market. After the original patent expires, patients have a more affordable choice in generic versions. Organisations devoted to consumer rights and protection may be interested in making sure that patients are informed about and protected when taking Viagra.

In conclusion, Viagra is a drug that involves a variety of parties, including pharmaceutical firms, medical professionals, and patients. These stakeholders' interests span a wide range of topics, including marketing, legislation, research, and patient care.

BIOLOGICAL FACTORS AFFECTING FEMALE VIAGRA

Female Viagra or other drugs intended to treat female sexual dysfunction may function differently depending on biological factors. The following are some significant biological variables that can impact the efficacy and response to such treatments:

Levels of hormones

Both male and female sexual health depend on hormonal balance. Variations in the levels of the hormones oestrogen and testosterone can affect a woman's level of sexual desire, arousal, and satisfaction. Sexual dysfunction can result from any disruptions or hormone imbalances.

Periodic Menstruation and Menopause

Sexual desire and arousal can be impacted by hormonal changes that occur during a woman's menstrual cycle and menopause. A drop in oestrogen levels during menopause can cause symptoms like dry vagina and a decreased libido.

Vascular Health and Blood Flow:

sufficient blood supply to the Genitalia are necessary for eliciting and enjoying sexual arousal. Sexual function can be impacted by any conditions that have an impact on blood circulation, such as diabetes or cardiovascular disease.

Physiological Action:

In order to respond sexually, the central nervous system is essential. Multiple sclerosis and other nerve-damaging diseases can make it difficult to feel arousal and pleasure during sexual activity. psychological elements

Sexual health is significantly influenced by psychological health. A woman's capacity to experience sexual arousal or pleasure in sexual activity can be significantly impacted by illnesses like anxiety, depression, or past trauma.

Drugs and Adverse Reactions:

Some drugs, including some birth control pills, antipsychotics, and antidepressants, can have side effects that interfere with sexual desire and function. Female Viagra or other treatments of a similar nature may be beneficial for women taking these medications minimise these outcomes.

Chronic Health Issues:

Sexual dysfunction in women can be exacerbated by longterm medical conditions like diabetes, hypertension, and autoimmune diseases. The balance of hormones, blood flow, and nerve function can all be impacted by these conditions.

Health in Reproduction:

Sexual function may change as a result of pregnancy, childbirth, and breastfeeding. Arousal and satisfaction issues may be exacerbated by hormonal changes and changes in the pelvic floor muscles.

Sexual Wellness: Sexual activity can be uncomfortable or painful due to conditions like vaginal atrophy, vulvodynia, or infections, which can then affect sexual desire. variations in anatomy

Sexual function may be impacted by differences in female genitalia anatomy. For instance, conditions like vaginismus, in which the vaginal muscles contract uncontrollably, can make penetration challenging or uncomfortable.

Ageing:

hormonal changes brought on by ageing, Health in general and blood flow can have an impact on sexual function. As women get older, it's typical for them to notice changes in their level of arousal and desire.

Lifestyle variables

Sexual dysfunction can be brought on by factors like smoking, binge drinking, and a sedentary lifestyle, which can all have an impact on blood flow, hormone balance, and general health.

Self-Esteem and Body Image:

A satisfying sexual relationship requires a positive body image and strong self-esteem. Inability to arouse and experience sexual pleasure can be caused by a negative body image or low self-esteem.

In order to increase sexual desire and satisfaction, female Viagra and related treatments for female sexual dysfunction address these biological factors. However, it's crucial to remember that sexual health is complicated and requires a comprehensive approach that takes relationship and psychological factors into account is often necessary for effective treatment. Consulting a healthcare provider who specializes in sexual health is essential for a comprehensive assessment and personalized treatment plan.

ADDYL

An FDA-approved drug called ADDYI (flibanserin) is used to treat premenopausal women with hypoactive sexual desire disorder (HSDD). Sexual desire that is persistently low or absent and causes distress or interpersonal issues is a defining feature of HSDD.

Here is a thorough explanation of ADDYI:

1. Mechanism of Action: Serotonin and dopamine are the two neurotransmitters that ADDYI specifically targets in the brain. It seeks to reestablish the equilibrium of these chemicals, which are thought to contribute to sexual desire.

2. Indications: Premenopausal females who experience

HSDD should take ADDYI. Both men and postmenopausal women are not intended users of this medication.

3. Clinical Trials: ADDYI was approved after undergoing extensive clinical tests to determine its safety and effectiveness. Studies showed that women taking ADDYI noticed an increase in breast size. decrease in low libidorelated distress and an increase in sexual desire.

4. Dosage and Administration: A dose of 100 mg taken once daily before bed is advised. It is crucial to adhere to the dosing schedule recommended by a healthcare professional.

5. Potential Side Effects: Common ADDYI side effects could include dry mouth, nausea, sleepiness, fatigue, and dizziness. Low blood pressure and loss of consciousness are uncommon but serious side effects, especially when combined with alcohol or certain medications.

6. Contraindications and Precautions: ADDYI should not

be used by people who have liver impairment or regularly consume alcohol. Because of the potentially harmful interactions, it shouldn't be used along with alcohol or specific medications. It's crucial to talk about any recent Before beginning ADDYI, discuss any medications or medical issues with a healthcare professional.

Alcohol Interaction: One of the important things to think about with ADDYI is how it interacts with alcohol. Alcohol consumption can cause a significant drop in blood pressure while taking ADDYI, which can be hazardous. Therefore, those who are taking ADDYI should completely avoid alcohol.

Effectiveness and Reaction: While some women with HSDD may find success with ADDYI, this is not always the case. Furthermore, it might take some time for a woman to detect an increase in her desire for sex. It's crucial to be patient and use the medication as prescribed by a healthcare professional.

9. Consultation with a Healthcare Professional: Women considering ADDYI should speak with a healthcare professional who can assess their particular situation and go over any potential advantages. and dangers, and decide whether ADDYI is the best course of action.

10. Regulatory Approval: After being initially rejected in

2010 due to worries about its efficacy and side effects, ADDYI received FDA approval in 2015.

11. Availability: ADDYI can only be purchased with a prescription from a doctor or an authorised pharmacy.

12. Patients who are prescribed ADDYI should receive thorough education about the medication, including instructions for use, possible side effects, and the value of abstaining from alcohol.

13. Follow-Up Care: It's essential to schedule routine follow-up appointments with a healthcare professional to assess the efficiency and safety of ADDYI as well as to address any worries or

inquiries.

VYLEESI

The U.S. Food and Drug Administration (FDA) has given the drug Vyleesi, also known by the generic name bremelanotide, approval to treat acquired, generalised hypoactive sexual desire disorder (HSDD) in premenopausal women. A persistent lack of interest in sexual activity that upsets others or interferes with relationships is a sign of HSDD. Here is a summary of Vyleesi:

1. Mechanism of Action: Melanocortin receptors, which are involved in arousing sexual desire, are stimulated by vyleesi. It is thought to open up neural pathways that improve sexual responsiveness and motivation.

2. Vyleesi is recommended for the treatment of HSDD in premenopausal females. Both men and postmenopausal women are not intended users of this medication.

3. Clinical Trials: Numerous clinical trials were conducted before Vyleesi was approved. its effectiveness and safety according to studies, women who took Vyleesi reported having more sexual desire and feeling less stress because of their low libido.

4. Dosage and Administration: Vyleesi is injected at least 45 minutes before the planned sexual activity, usually into the thigh or abdomen. The medication should only be used once within a 24-hour period and should only be taken as needed.

5. Potential Side Effects: Vyleesi frequently causes headaches, flushing, and nausea. Most of the time, these side effects are minor and transient. It's crucial to adhere to the dosage recommendations and avoid exceeding them.

6. Vyleesi is contraindicated in people with uncontrolled hypertension (high blood pressure), according to the warnings and precautions listed in point six such as heart disease.

Combining it with drugs or other substances that lower blood pressure is not advised. A healthcare professional should evaluate the patient's cardiovascular health before prescribing Vyleesi.

7. Effectiveness and Response: As with any medication, Vyleesi may have different effects on different people. It might help some women with HSDD, but it might not help everyone. Patients should discuss the effectiveness of their medication and any side effects they may be experiencing with their doctor.

8. Regulatory Approval: In June 2019, the FDA gave its blessing to Vyleesi. It was introduced as an alternative form of treatment for premenopausal women with HSDD.

9. Consultation with a Healthcare Professional: Women considering Vyleesi should speak with a healthcare professional who can assess their unique situation, go over potential advantages, and explain any risks and decide if Vyleesi is a suitable course of treatment.

10. Vyleesi is only available with a prescription and must be obtained from a healthcare professional.

11. Patients who are prescribed Vyleesi should receive thorough education about the drug, including instructions for use, possible side effects, and any necessary precautions. Additionally, they should be urged to tell their doctor about any additional medications they are taking.

12. Follow-Up Care: It's critical to schedule routine follow-up visits with a healthcare professional to discuss any concerns and track the effectiveness and safety of Vyleesi.

CHAPTER FOUR

Combination of Viagra with other medications and alcohol

Combination with other medications :

Nitroglycerin and nitrates

When using Viagra, one of the most important things to keep in mind is how it will interact with nitrates, a class of drugs frequently prescribed for angina (chest pain). Together, nitrates and Viagra can cause a significant drop in blood pressure and, in some cases, a life-threatening situation because they both widen blood vessels.

Beta-Blockers

Alpha-blockers are drugs that are prescribed to treat benign prostatic hyperplasia (enlarged prostate) and high blood pressure (hypertension). Additionally, they can cause a drop in blood pressure when taken with Viagra. If these medications must be taken together, medical professionals must carefully monitor the dosages.

Additional ED medications

Other drugs, like tadalafil, are prescribed to treat ED (Levitra) and vardenafil (Cialis). Combining these with Viagra may increase the chance of side effects while offering little additional help for better erectile function. 2.4 Drugs with antifungal and antibiotic properties

Antifungal and antibiotic medications can affect how Viagra is metabolised in the body, potentially increasing the amount of the drug in the blood. The likelihood of complications and side effects may increase as a result.

HIV Protease Inhibitors

Viagra levels may rise in the body when combined with protease inhibitors, a class of drugs used to treat HIV. This might exacerbate side effects and necessitate changing the dosage.

COMBINING VIAGRA AND ALCOHOL

Alcohol and Sexual Function

Alcohol is a central nervous system depressant, and its effects on sexual function can be complex:

•   Moderate Consumption: In some cases, a small amount of alcohol can help reduce anxiety and inhibitions, which may contribute to improved sexual performance and desire.

•   Excessive Consumption: Excessive alcohol consumption can lead to impaired sexual function, including difficulty achieving or maintaining an erection (alcohol-induced erectile dysfunction).

Interaction with Blood Pressure

Both Viagra and alcohol can lower blood pressure, and combining the two can intensify this effect. A significant drop in blood pressure can lead to dizziness, lightheadedness, and in severe cases, loss of consciousness.

Impaired Judgment and Reflexes

Alcohol impairs judgment, coordination, and reflexes. Combining Viagra with alcohol can potentially lead to risky sexual behavior, accidents, and reduced ability to respond to emergency situations.

Potential Impact on Viagra's Effectiveness

Alcohol can delay the onset of Viagra's effects and potentially reduce its effectiveness. It may take longer to achieve an erection, or the effects may be less pronounced when alcohol is present in the system.

Safety Concerns

The combination of Viagra and alcohol can increase the risk of side effects such as headache, dizziness, flushing, and gastrointestinal discomfort.

RECOMMENDATIONS AND PRECAUTIONS

Healthcare Provider Guidance

Individuals considering the use of Viagra in combination with alcohol should consult their healthcare provider. A healthcare professional can assess their specific health status and provide personalized advice.

Safe Alcohol Consumption

If a healthcare provider permits the consumption of alcohol while using Viagra, it should be done in moderation. This typically means limiting alcohol intake to one or two standard drinks.

Monitoring for Side Effects

Individuals combining Viagra and alcohol should be vigilant for any unusual side effects and promptly report them to their healthcare provider.

Avoiding Self-Medication

Self-medicating with Viagra or obtaining it from unofficial or unregulated sources is strongly discouraged. This can lead to incorrect dosages, increased risks, and potential harm.

Seeking Immediate Medical Attention

In the event of severe side effects or a prolonged and painful erection (priapism), individuals should seek immediate medical attention.

Conclusion

The combination of Viagra and alcohol should be approached with caution. While Viagra can be an effective treatment for ED, the use of both substances should prioritize safety and adherence to healthcare provider recommendations. Open communication with a healthcare provider is essential to ensure that any potential risks are minimized, and the benefits of the medication are maximized

Alcohol and Sexual Performance

Alcohol is a depressant that can have an impact on the brain's nervous system, which is essential for arousing sexual desire. Chronic erectile dysfunction or even temporary erectile dysfunction can result from excessive alcohol use.

Interaction with Blood Pressure

Alcohol and Viagra both lower blood pressure. When the two are combined, the blood pressure can drop significantly, which can be hazardous and even fatal.

IMPAIRMENT OF REFLEXES AND JUDGEMENT

Decision-making and coordination may be affected by alcohol. Alcohol and Viagra may cause erratic sexual behaviour or accidents because of slow reflexes.

Advice and Safety Measures

Advice for Healthcare Providers

Anyone thinking about taking Viagra with other drugs or alcohol should speak to their doctor first. To offer individualised guidance, a healthcare professional can evaluate a patient's health status, medications, and lifestyle choices.

Legal Liquor Consumption

If your doctor permits you to drink alcohol while taking Viagra, it's important to do so sparingly. Typically, this means having no more than one or two standard drinks.

Monitoring for Adverse Reactions

When taking Viagra with other medications, users should be on the lookout for any unusual side effects and notify their doctor right away.

Refusing to Self-Medicate

It is strongly advised against using Viagra for selfmedication or getting it from unreliable or unapproved sources. Inappropriate dosages, elevated risks, and potential harm can result from this.

Seeking Right Away Medical Care

It's critical to seek immediate medical attention if you experience serious side effects like a sudden drop in blood pressure or a protracted, painful erection (priapism).

Summary

The When taking Viagra along with other medications and alcohol, you should seek professional advice. Viagra can be a very successful treatment for erectile dysfunction, but when using it, caution and adherence to medical professional advice should always come first. To ensure that any potential risks are reduced and the therapeutic benefits   of   the   medication are   maximised,   open communication with a healthcare professional is essential.

INTERACTION OF VIAGRA WITH NITRATE

Due to potential fatal consequences, the interaction between Viagra (sildenafil) and nitrates must be carefully considered and avoided. A class of drugs known as nitrates is frequently prescribed to treat angina (chest pain) and specific heart conditions. The following justifies why taking Viagra with nitrates is hazardous:

1. Action Mechanism:

Phosphodiesterase type 5 (PDE5) inhibitor, Viagra (Sildenafil). It functions by widening blood vessels throughout the body, especially those in the genital region, to improve blood flow and aid in achieving and maintaining an erection.

Nitrates: To relax and enlarge blood vessels, nitrates like nitroglycerin, isosorbide dinitrate, and isosorbide mononitrate are frequently used. They are recommended to treat chest pain brought on by inadequate blood supply to the heart muscle.

2. The Hypotension Risk:

The main risk of taking Viagra and nitrates together is the possibility of developing severe hypotension (low blood pressure). Nitrates and Viagra both have their own effects on blood vessel expansion and blood pressure reduction. These effects may combine to cause a significant drop in blood pressure when combined.

3. Potential Repercussions

Lightheadedness, fainting, and loss of consciousness are all symptoms of low blood pressure. This can be particularly hazardous if it happens while driving or performing other tasks that call for alertness.

Heart Health: Taking Viagra and nitrates together can strain the heart. This may be fatal for people who already have heart problems.

The interaction may also result in additional side effects, such as nausea, vertigo, and blurred vision in extreme circumstances, a heart attack.

4. Important Safety Measures:

Before considering using Viagra, people who take nitrates should tell their doctor about the medication.

To avoid prescribing Viagra to people taking nitrates, healthcare professionals should thoroughly review a patient's medical history.

Instructions for the safe and responsible use of medications should be followed by patients by their doctor.

5. ED Alternatives:

If someone is experiencing erectile dysfunction and is worried about how nitrates will interact with their angina or heart condition, they should talk to their doctor about other ED treatments. In such circumstances, a number of alternative treatments might be safer and more appropriate.

In conclusion, because of the potential for a severe drop in blood pressure, it is not advised to take Viagra with nitrates like nitroglycerin the resulting high blood pressure. This interaction should be avoided at all costs because it may be fatal. Consult your doctor to discuss safer alternatives for the treatment of erectile dysfunction if you have angina, heart disease, or are taking nitrates. When considering the use of medications, safety should always come first, especially when they interact with other prescribed medications.

VIAGRA EFFECTS AND OTHER DRUGS

1.1 Inhibition of Phosphodiesterase Type 5 (PDE5)

Viagra works by preventing the PDE5 enzyme from dissolving cyclic guanosine monophosphate (cGMP). This allows for increased blood flow to the penis and facilitates an erection by extending the effects of cGMP.

PART 2: NITRATE INTERACTIONS 2.1.1 NITRATES FOR ANGINA

It is not advised to combine Viagra with nitrates (such as nitroglycerin). Both medications cause vasodilation, which lowers blood pressure to a potentially hazardous level. This interaction may cause fainting, wooziness, or, in extreme cases, hypotension that is life-threatening.

3.1 Alpha-Blockers for Hypertension (Part 3: Alpha-Blockers and Viagra)

When combining Viagra with alpha-blockers (such as doxazosin) to treat hypertension, caution is advised. Both drugs can lower blood pressure, and their combined use could have an adverse effect excessive blood pressure decline. Close monitoring and appropriate dosage adjustments are crucial.

PART 4: INTERACTIONS BETWEEN ANTIFUNGALS AND ANTIBIOTICS

4.1 Antifungal Azole

Itraconazole and ketoconazole, for example, can inhibit the metabolism of Viagra, resulting in elevated blood levels. The effects and potential side effects of Viagra may be exacerbated by this.

4.2 Antibiotics with Macrolides

Antibiotics called macrolides, such as erythromycin and clarithromycin, can also prevent the body from metabolising Viagra. When these medications are taken together, the body may produce more Viagra, which could amplify its effects and side effects.

Protease inhibitors for HIV (Part 5)

HIV medication interactions, section 5.1

Ritonavir and indinavir, two protease inhibitors used to treat HIV, can raise the blood levels of Viagra. It may be necessary to adjust the dosage and keep a close eye out for this interaction possible negative effects.

PART 6: ADVERSE EFFECTS FROM OTHER ED DRUGS
6.1 Viagra and Other PDE5 Inhibitors Together

It is generally not advised to combine Viagra with other PDE5 inhibitors (such as tadalafil or vardenafil) because doing so can increase the risk of side effects without necessarily improving erectile function.

SSRIs and SNRIs in Part 7

7.1 Viagra and antidepressants

Serotonin-norepinephrine reuptake inhibitors (SNRIs) and selective serotonin reuptake inhibitors (SSRIs) can have an impact on sexual function. In some situations, combining these medications with Viagra may be an option, but it must be carefully evaluated and monitored for possible interactions.

PART 8: ADDITIONAL IDEAS

8.1 Supplements and over-the-counter medicines made from herbs

Over-the-counter medicines and some herbal supplements may interact with Viagra. It's critical to let medical professionals know about all substances being taken, including over-the-counter medicines.

PART 9: FINAL VERDICT

For safe and effective use, it is essential to comprehend the potential interactions between Viagra and other medications. In analysing unique patient profiles, making tailored recommendations, and ensuring that any potential risks are minimised, healthcare providers play a crucial role. When combining Viagra with other medications, open communication with a healthcare professional is essential to getting the best results.

AN DETAILED INVESTIGATION OF SEXUAL

Dysfunction Medication

Sexual dysfunction is a widespread problem that affects people of all sexes and ages. Thankfully, there are many medications that can treat sexual dysfunction. We will explore the conditions they treat, their mechanisms of action, potential side effects, and considerations for use as we delve into the world of sexual dysfunction medications in this thorough guide.

1.1 Understanding Sexual Dysfunction 1. Introduction to Sexual Dysfunction Medication

The term "sexual dysfunction" refers to a wide range of problems that make it difficult for someone to enjoy themselves during sex or to engage in satisfying sexual activity. Erectile dysfunction (ED), female sexual dysfunction, early ejaculation, and hypoactive sexual desire disorder (HSDD) are examples of common sexual dysfunctions. These conditions may be brought on by relational, psychological, or physical issues.

1.2 The Function of Medicines

The treatment of sexual dysfunction involves the use of medications significantly. They can deal with the physiological or psychological causes of these conditions. The treatments for each type of sexual dysfunction will be discussed in this manual along with their mechanisms of action, potential side effects, and usage guidelines.

2. Erectile dysfunction medications

Erectile a common sexual dysfunction in men is erection dysfunction (ED), which is defined as the inability to obtain or maintain an erection strong enough for sexual activity. There are numerous medications available to treat ED.

2.1 Viagra (sildenafil)

One of the most popular treatments for ED is the drug sildenafil, sold under the brand name Viagra. It functions by improving blood flow to the penis and is typically taken as needed.

2.2 Cialis (tadalafil)

Since Tadalafil, also known as Cialis, takes longer to take effect than Viagra, sexual activity can be more spontaneous.

2.3 Levitra (vardenafil)

Levitra, which is sold as vardenafil, works similarly to Viagra. ED is also treated with it on an as-needed basis.

2.4: Avanafil (Stendra) :Avanafil, sold under the brand name Stendra, is a more recent ED drug with a reputation for acting quickly—often within 15 minutes.

2.5: Alprostadil

Alprostadil is a medication that can be used topically, intravenously, or as a suppository to treat erection problems.

TREATMENT WITH TESTOSTERONE REPLACEMENT

Insufficient testosterone can contribute to ED. When low testosterone is found to be the root of erectile dysfunction, testosterone replacement therapy is an option.

3. Drugs for treating female erectile dysfunction

Complex issues like desire, arousal, and pain can all play a role in female sexual dysfunction. Specific facets of female sexual dysfunction can be treated with medication.

3. Flibanserin (Addyi)

Flibanserin, also known as Addyi, is approved to treat premenopausal women with hypoactive sexual desire disorder (HSDD). targeting the brain's neurotransmitters increasing sexual desire in the brain.

3.2 Bremelanotide (Vyleesi),

Premenopausal women with acquired, generalised hypoactive sexual desire disorder (HSDD) can be treated with the injectable medication bremelanotide, which is marketed under the brand name Vyleesi. It causes a number of brain receptors related to sexual motivation and responsiveness to become active.

3.3.3 Hormone Treatment

When female sex dysfunction is brought on by hormonal imbalances, such as low oestrogen levels during menopause, hormone therapy may be an option.

4. Premature Ejaculation Medicines

Men frequently experience premature ejaculation (PE), and medications can help prolong the ejaculation period.

4.1   Dapoxetine

Premature ejaculation is the only condition for which dapoxetine has been given specific approval. It is an SSRI, or selective serotonin reuptake inhibitor, and it can postpone ovulation.

4.2   Sertraline

Another SSRI, sertraline, has been utilised off-label to treat early ejaculation by postponing it.

4.3   Topical Painkillers

There are several types of topical anaesthetics, such as creams and sprays, that can be used to lessen penile sensitivity and lengthen the time until ejaculation.

5. Drugs used to treat Hypoactive Sexual Desire Disorder (HSDD)

A persistent lack of sexual desire is a symptom of hypoactive sexual desire disorder (HSDD). There are numerous medications that can be used to treat it.

(Addyi) Flibanserin

For premenopausal women with HSDD, flibanserin, also known as Addyi, has been approved. It increases sexual desire by interacting with serotonin and dopamine receptors.

5.2: Bremelanotide (Vyleesi), For premenopausal women with HSDD, there is also bremelanotide, marketed under the brand name Vyleesi. To increase sexual motivation and responsiveness, it works by targeting melanocortin receptors in the brain.

6. Typical Side Effects and Things to Think About

6.1 Adverse Effects of ED Drugs

Drugs for ED can cause negative side effects like headaches, flushing, nasal congestion, and digestive problems. One uncommon but severe side effect is priapism, which causes an extended and painful erection. 6.2 Drugs for Female Sexual Dysfunction: Side Effects

Dizziness, nausea, and fatigue are common side effects of medications for female sexual dysfunction. They may interact if taken with alcohol or specific medications.

6.3 Negative Effects of Premature Ejaculation Drugs

When used for early ejaculation, SSRIs can have negative side effects like nausea, vertigo, and decreased libido. Topical anaesthetics could make you less sensitive during sex.

6.4 Drugs for HSDD: Adverse Reactions

Dizziness, nausea, and fatigue may be side effects of HSDD medications. Interactions between these medications and alcohol can occur.

6.5 Medication Use Considerations Information about current medications, discussion of potential drug interactions, and adherence to recommended dosages are all factors in safe and effective medication use.

7. Doppler Effects of Potential Drugs

7.1 Nitrate-Medication Interactions

Due to a significant drop in blood pressure, taking ED medications, particularly Viagra, with nitrates for chest pain is risky.

interaction with alpha-blockers,

Alpha-blockers prescribed for hypertension and ED medications may interact, lowering blood pressure. Combining these medications necessitates changing the dosage.

7.3: Interactions with Other Medications, Section

The effectiveness and safety of ED medications may be impacted by interactions with other medications, including antifungals, antibiotics, and HIV medications.

8. Over-the-Counter and Herbal Treatments

8.1 Yohimbe

A herbal supplement called yohimbe has been used to treat ED. Although it can cause serious side effects and should only be used under strict supervision.

8.2 L-Arginine

Due to its potential to increase blood flow, the amino acid L-arginine is frequently promoted as a natural treatment for ED. Its effectiveness is still being studied.

8.3 Gingko Biloba

The effectiveness of the herbal supplement ginkgo biloba for treating ED is not well known, but it may enhance blood flow and cognitive function.

8.4 DHEA: The hormone DHEA, which is produced by the adrenal glands, is occasionally marketed as a treatment for ED. However, there is little scientific data to back up its use.

9.   Consultations and Evaluation

   9.1   The Function of Healthcare Professionals

Medical professionals are crucial in identifying and treating sexual dysfunction. They can also suggest suitable medical interventions, such as drugs.

   9.2   Relationship and Psychological Factors Psychological and interpersonal dynamics can significantly exacerbate sexual dysfunction. When planning a treatment, healthcare professionals frequently take these factors into account.

   9.3   Individualised Treatment Programmes

Each patient's unique needs and concerns should be taken into account when providing treatment for sexual dysfunction. For the development of individualised treatment plans, a thorough assessment is necessary.

10. Responsibility and Safety in Medication Use

10.1 The Importance of Prescription Drugs To ensure quality, safety, and efficacy, prescription drugs should only be obtained from authorised healthcare professionals.

10.2 Safe Medication Use

Adhering to dosage guidelines, being aware of potential side effects, and avoiding alcohol or other substances that might interact with the medication are all necessary for safe medication use.

10.3 Consistent Check-Ins and Monitoring

It's crucial to schedule routine follow-up appointments with medical professionals to assess the efficiency and security of the drug. Depending on each person's response, adjustments might be required.

11. Finalization

The quality of life for those who suffer from sexual dysfunction can be significantly improved by medications, which are essential in treating the condition. Making educated decisions about treatment requires an understanding of the various options available, their mechanisms of action, potential side effects, and considerations for use. Developing individualized treatment plans that address the needs of each patient requires close collaboration with healthcare professionals and a thorough assessment.

1. Introduction to High Blood Pressure and Antihypertensive Drugs

1.1 Knowledge of Hypertension

A chronic medical condition called hypertension, also known as high blood pressure, is characterized by elevated artery blood pressure levels. It is a significant risk factor for kidney disease, vascular disorders, and other illnesses like heart attacks, strokes, and cardiovascular diseases.

Antihypertensive Medications

1.2 The Function of Antihypertensive Drugs

A key element of controlling hypertension is the use of antihypertensive medications. They assist in lowering blood pressure, decreasing the chance of complications, and enhancing cardiovascular health in general. The various classes of antihypertensive medications, their mechanisms of action, potential side effects, and variables influencing their use will all be covered in this guide.

2.   Altering Your Lifestyle and Non-Pharmacological

Methods

2.1 Nutrition and Diet

Dietary changes are essential role in blood pressure regulation. Reducing sodium intake, eating more foods high in potassium, and following the DASH (Dietary Approaches to Stop Hypertension) diet are all advised.

Physical Exercise

Lower blood pressure is linked to regular physical activity. We'll talk about the suggested exercise regimens and how physical fitness affects hypertension.

2.3 Stress Reduction

Blood pressure that is too high can be caused by stress. We'll look at methods for reducing stress like mindfulness, meditation, and relaxation exercises.

2.4 Quitting Smoking

An important risk factor for hypertension is smoking. We'll look at smoking's effects on blood pressure as well as methods for quitting.

2.5 Consumption of alcohol

Alcoholism in excess can result in hypertension. Guidelines for responsible alcohol consumption and the connection between alcohol and heart rate.

3. Antihypertensive Drug Class Categories

The various drug classes that make up antihypertensive medications each have unique mechanisms of action. We'll look at the following categories:

3 Diuretics

Diuretics encourage the body to expel extra water and sodium, which in turn reduces blood volume and lowers blood pressure.

Beta Blockers

Beta-blockers lower blood pressure and lessen the workload placed on the heart by lowering heart rate and the force with which it contracts.

ACE Inhibitors, 3.3%

Angiotensin-converting enzyme (ACE) inhibitors cause blood vessels to dilate and lower blood pressure by preventing the production of angiotensin II, a potent vasoconstrictor.

3.4 ARBs, or angiotensin II receptor blockers

By attaching to angiotensin II receptors, ARBs stop the hormone's action, causing blood vessels to widen and blood pressure to drop.

Calcium channel blockers (CCBs), or 3.5 restrict the entry of calcium into smooth muscle cells, which relaxes and dilates blood vessels and lowers blood pressure.

3.6 Beta-Blockers

Norepinephrine's action is inhibited by alpha-blockers, which causes blood vessels to widen and blood pressure to drop.

3.7 Alpha-Beta Preventatives

Alpha-beta blockers lower blood pressure and heart rate by combining the effects of alpha- and beta-blockers.

Renin Inhibitors 3.8

Renin inhibitors work by inhibiting the renin-angiotensin system, which reduces the production of angiotensin I and angiotensin II and lowers blood pressure by widening blood vessels.

Vasodilators

Vasodilators cause dilation and a drop in blood pressure by relaxing the smooth muscle in blood vessel walls.

3.10 Acting Central Agents

The central nervous system is affected by central acting agents, which lessen blood vessel constriction and lower blood pressure.

4. Action Mechanisms medications for treating hypertension Understanding how antihypertensive medications lower blood pressure requires knowledge of their mechanisms of action. We will delve into each drug class's mechanisms of action, including how they impact blood vessel tone, heart rate, and blood volume.

5. Adjuvant Therapy

To achieve blood pressure control, it is frequently necessary to combine antihypertensive medications. We will examine the justification for combination therapy and typical drug combinations, as well as their advantages and drawbacks.

6. Side Effects and Antihypertensive Drug Considerations

6.1 Typical Adverse Effects

Dizziness, fatigue, and electrolyte imbalances are a few of the side effects that antihypertensive medications can produce. We'll talk about the side effects connected to various drug classes.

6.2 Serious Adverse Reactions

Antihypertensive medications can occasionally cause serious side effects, such as angioedema, kidney problems, and electrolyte problems. These harmful side effects will be described, along with how to handle them.

6.3 Special Populations Considerations

Antihypertensive therapies must be individually tailored for special populations, such as women who are pregnant and people with particular medical conditions. We'll look at these groups' considerations.

6.4.2 Drug Interactions

The effectiveness and safety of antihypertensive medications may be impacted by interactions with other medications. We will look at typical drug interactions and management techniques for them. 6.5 Adherence and Compliance

For effective blood pressure control, compliance and adherence to antihypertensive medication regimens are essential. We'll talk about ways to increase medication adherence.

7. Blood Pressure Target Levels and Monitoring

7.1 Home Blood Pressure Monitoring Monitoring your blood pressure at home is a useful tool for monitoring changes in your blood pressure over time visits to healthcare providers. We will look at its advantages and ideal procedures.

Office Blood Pressure Measurements, Section 7.2

For diagnosis and treatment choices, the accuracy of blood pressure measurements taken in the office is essential.
We'll talk about how to measure things properly.

7.3 Objective Blood Pressure Ranges

For various patient populations, guidelines recommend specific target blood pressure levels. These target levels and their clinical relevance will be discussed.

8. The significance of blood pressure management Eliminating Cardiovascular Risk

Heart attacks and strokes are significantly decreased in risk thanks to effective blood pressure management.

8.2 Preventing Organ Damage to the Target

Vital organs like the heart, kidneys, and blood vessels can suffer damage from hypertension. Controlling blood pressure is crucial for avoiding this harm.

8.3 Improving General Health and Well-Being Maintaining a healthy blood pressure level helps with better general health, which includes increased longevity and life quality.

9. Finalization

A key component of managing hypertension is the use of antihypertensive medications. Controlling blood pressure is essential for lowering cardiovascular risk, avoiding damage to target organs, and enhancing general health and wellbeing. The various classes of antihypertensive medications, their mechanisms of action, potential side effects, and usage considerations are all covered in detail in this extensive guide, along with the significance of nonpharmacological methods and blood pressure monitoring.

SUPPLEMENTS AND VIAGRA HERBS AND VIAGRA

Supplements and herbs are often promoted as natural

alternatives or complementary treatments for erectile dysfunction (ED), for which Viagra (sildenafil) is a wellknown prescription medication. While some supplements and herbs may have anecdotal or limited scientific evidence suggesting they could help with ED, it's important to exercise caution and consult with a healthcare professional before using them. Here's an overview of some supplements and herbs that have been associated with potential benefits for ED:

1. **L-arginine**: L-arginine is an amino acid that may help relax blood vessels, leading to improved blood flow. Some studies suggest that it might be beneficial for ED. However, it can interact with certain medications, so it's crucial to talk to your doctor before using it.

2. Ginseng: Commonly used herbs with potential benefits for ED include Korean red ginseng and Panax ginseng. Although some studies have found benefits, more studies are required to confirm their effectiveness.

3. Epimedium: is also known as horny goat weed, is a herb that is thought to function similarly to Viagra by enhancing blood flow to the penis. There isn't much data to back up its effectiveness, though.

4. Maca Root: A plant called maca has been traditionally used to improve sexual performance. More research is required, but some studies indicate it might help ED.

5. Yohimbe: This supplement, which is sometimes used to treat ED, is made from the bark of an African tree. However, it may cause adverse reactions and interact with other medications, so

Tribulus Terrestris: This herb is sometimes used for its potential to boost testosterone levels. Some studies have suggested it may have a modest benefit for ED.

It's important to note that the effectiveness and safety of these supplements and herbs can vary widely, and their use should be discussed with a healthcare provider.

Additionally, you should never use them as a substitute for prescribed medications like Viagra without consulting a doctor. Viagra is a well-researched and regulated medication, while supplements and herbs may not have the same level of scientific scrutiny or quality control.

Always consult with a healthcare professional before trying any supplement or herbal remedy for ED, and remember that lifestyle factors such as maintaining a healthy diet, regular exercise, managing stress, and avoiding smoking and excessive alcohol consumption can also have a significant impact on erectile function.

VIAGRA AND VITAMIN

Even though Viagra isn't a vitamin, maintaining general health through a balanced diet that includes vitamins and minerals can help with sexual health. Several vitamins and minerals are crucial for both general health and sexual well-being, such as:

Vitamin D: Healthy levels of vitamin D are linked to improved sexual performance. Vitamin D can be obtained from the sun, specific foods, and supplements.

Vitamin C: An antioxidant, vitamin C can enhance blood circulation, which is good for sexual health. Fruits and vegetables contain it.

Niacin, a form of vitamin B3, may improve erectile function by increasing blood flow. It is present in nuts, fish, and meat.

Vitamin E: An antioxidant, vitamin E can aid in enhancing cardiovascular health, which is crucial for sexual function. Nuts, seeds, and vegetable oils contain it.

Zinc: Zinc is a mineral that is crucial for the production of testosterone and general sexual health. Meat, dairy products, and some nuts contain it.

When possible, it's best to obtain these vitamins and minerals through a healthy diet. However, it's advisable to speak with a healthcare provider if you think you may have particular deficiencies or health issues. They can evaluate your specific requirements and may suggest vitamin or mineral supplements, but it's important to use supplements only when directed by a doctor because an excessive intake of them can have negative effects.

FOOD AND VIAGRA INTERACTIONS

How quickly and effectively Viagra (sildenafil) works in your body may be influenced by the foods you eat. These interactions must be understood because they may affect the medication's efficacy and safety. Here are some important things to think about in relation to Viagra and food interactions.

Despite the fact that vitamins and minerals can improve general health and if you have been prescribed Viagra for erectile dysfunction, they might not be able to take the place of that medication. For the management of your medical condition, always abide by your doctor's recommendations.

1. Fatty Foods: Eating a lot of fat right before taking Viagra can prevent it from being absorbed into the bloodstream. Fatty foods may slow down the rate of sildenafil absorption in the body, delaying the onset of the drug's effects. For quicker and more reliable results, it is advised to take Viagra on an empty stomach or with a meal low in fat.
2. Grapefruit and Grapefruit Juice: Grapefruit and grapefruit juice both contain substances that may affect how Viagra and other medications are metabolized by your body. Increased blood levels of sildenafil due to this interaction could increase the risk of adverse effects. While taking Viagra, it is best to stay away from grapefruit and grapefruit juice.
3. Alcohol: While a small amount of alcohol may not affect Viagra directly, excessive alcohol use can make it harder to achieve and keep an erection. Additionally, it can raise the

possibility of adverse effects like low blood pressure and dizziness. If you intend to use Viagra, it's best to only drink occasionally.

4. Meals that are heavy or spicy may also slow down the absorption of Viagra in addition to fatty foods. A substantial, spicy meal may cause the effects of the medication to take longer to take effect.

5. Empty Stomach: Take Viagra on an empty stomach for the fastest onset of action. This indicates that you should wait at least two hours to eat before taking the medication.

It's crucial to talk to your doctor about any worries or queries you may have about Viagra and food interactions. Based on your unique needs and circumstances, they can offer tailored advice. Always adhere to your doctor's dosage recommendations, and never alter the timing or dosage of Viagra without consulting them first. As a prescription drug, Viagra must be taken exactly as prescribed to achieve the best and safest results.

LAB TESTING AND VIAGRA

Sildenafil, the active ingredient in Viagra, is frequently prescribed without the need for laboratory testing. However, when determining whether a patient is a candidate for Viagra or when looking into the underlying causes of erectile dysfunction, healthcare professionals may order specific tests or assessments.

These tests can assist in confirming that Viagra is a suitable and safe treatment option.

Here are some situations in which lab testing or assessments may be considered:

1. Examining your physical condition and taking a thorough medical history are usually the first steps taken by your healthcare provider. This can aid in locating any underlying medical issues or danger signs that might be linked to erectile dysfunction.

2. Viagra has an impact on blood flow, so your doctor may

perform a cardiovascular health check. To make sure your heart is healthy, tests like blood pressure readings, lipid analyses, and electrocardiograms (ECGs) may be performed.

3. Hormone Levels: A blood test to measure hormone levels, including testosterone, may be advised in some circumstances, particularly if there are symptoms of hormonal problems.

4. Blood glucose testing may be advised by your doctor if diabetes is suspected as the root cause of erectile dysfunction (ED).

5. Psychological Evaluation: A psychologist or psychiatrist may be consulted to evaluate the psychological aspects of erectile dysfunction if psychological factors are suspected.

6. Drug Interactions: To make sure there are no Viagra contraindications or harmful interactions, your healthcare provider may ask about any other medications you are currently taking.

It's crucial to keep in mind that Viagra requires a prescription and that using it should only be done with a doctor's approval. Before recommending Viagra, they will take into account your medical history, general health, and any possible risk factors. In order to ensure your safety and rule out any underlying medical conditions that might call for particular treatment, lab tests and assessments are used. It's critical to speak with a healthcare professional if you have questions about erectile dysfunction or are considering taking Viagra either have inquiries about erectile dysfunction or are thinking about using Viagra.

THC AND CANNABIS INTERACTIONS WITH VIAGRA

When combined with Viagra (sildenafil), THC (tetrahydrocannabinol) and cannabis may cause interactions and side effects. It is essential to be aware of these interactions and to proceed with caution because they may affect the potency and security of both drugs.

1.THC and Viagra both have the ability to lower blood

pressure. When combined, they might have an additive effect that could result in dangerously low blood pressure, lightheadedness, fainting, and other negative side effects. It's crucial to monitor your blood pressure if you use Viagra and cannabis, especially if you take them both at the same time, and to get medical help if you experience symptoms of low blood pressure.

2. Viagra has cardiovascular side effects and is frequently prescribed to people who have underlying cardiovascular problems. When combined with Viagra, cannabis, especially when smoked, may cause an increase in heart rate and possibly increase the risk of heart-related complications. Heart disease sufferers should exercise extra caution.

3. Both substances have the potential to have negative side effects, including headache, dizziness, and changes in vision. Combining them may make these side effects more noticeable and less enjoyable.

4. Interaction with Other Medications: THC or cannabis use may interact with other medications you are taking if you also take Viagra. In order to receive safe and effective treatment, you should always let your healthcare provider know about all the medications you take.

5. Individual Reactions: Since everyone responds differently to the combination of Viagra and cannabis, it's important to pay attention to how you feel and speak with a doctor if you have any concerns.

It is advised to speak with a healthcare provider before combining Viagra and cannabis due to the possibility of interactions and the complexity of individual responses. Based on your unique medical needs and history, they can offer tailored advice. Healthcare professionals may occasionally advise against consuming both drugs at once, especially if you have specific medical conditions or are taking other medications.

When using these substances, it's crucial to prioritise your health and safety, and open communication with a healthcare provider is essential for helping you make knowledgeable decisions about their use.

INTERACTIONS BETWEEN VIAGRA AND CERTAIN MEDICAL CONDITIONS

Sildenafil, the active ingredient in Viagra, may interact with some medical conditions, potentially leading to complications or contraindications. Before taking Viagra, it is critical to let your doctor know about your medical history and any existing conditions. The following medical conditions could affect how Viagra works.

1. Viagra affects blood flow and can lower blood pressure, which are cardiovascular conditions. If you have a history of heart disease, angina (chest pain), arrhythmias (irregular heartbeats), or if you've recently experienced a heart attack or stroke, you should proceed with caution. Whether it is safe for you to take Viagra should be discussed with your healthcare provider.
2. Hypotension (Low Blood Pressure): Using Viagra may exacerbate this effect and result in dangerously low blood pressure, which could cause fainting, dizziness, or even a heart attack in people with low blood pressure that is already abnormally low or who are taking blood pressure-lowering medications.
3. Viagra is metabolised by the liver, so people with liver impairment may experience a slower breakdown of the drug, which could result in more side effects. In addition, kidney disease can hinder the body's ability to eliminate Viagra.
4. Eye Conditions: Using Viagra may increase your risk of experiencing side effects that affect your vision if you have certain eye conditions, such as retinitis pigmentosa or non-arteritic anterior ischemic optic neuropathy (NAION). Tell your doctor about any eye conditions you may have.

5. Stomach Ulcers: Viagra can cause gastrointestinal irritation, so it's important to talk to your doctor if you have a history of stomach ulcers or bleeding disorders.
6. Peyronie's Disease: Since Viagra has the potential to make Peyronie's disease, which is characterised by the curvature of the penis, worse, it may not be appropriate for people with this condition.
7. Sickle Cell Anaemia: People with sickle cell anaemia may experience priapism, a protracted and painful erection, more frequently when taking Viagra.
8. Leukaemia and multiple myeloma: Using Viagra may increase the risk of priapism in these diseases.
9. Anatomical Deformities or Penile Implants: Some anatomical deformities or penile implants may affect how well Viagra works.
10. Allergies: You shouldn't take Viagra if you are allergic to sildenafil or any of the other ingredients in it.
11. Current Medications: Be sure to let your doctor know about all of your current medications, including over-the-counter medicines, as Viagra may interact with a number of them, including nitrates (used to treat heart conditions), alphablockers, and some antifungal and HIV drugs.

Given your medical history, your healthcare provider is the best person to determine whether Viagra is right for you. To ensure your safety and the efficacy of the medication, they can advise you on possible interactions, alter dosages, or suggest different treatments if necessary.

PROBLEMS WITH THE LIVER OR KIDNEYS

1. Liver Issues:

- Liver disease: If you have a severe case of liver disease, your liver may not be able to effectively metabolise Viagra. This may lead to higher blood levels of the medication, which could raise the possibility of negative side effects. Your doctor might need to change the dosage or suggest different therapies depending on how severe your liver disease is.

- Hepatitis: Liver function may be impaired in some hepatitis patients. Your healthcare provider will need to know about your hepatitis status in order to determine whether Viagra is a safe option for you.

2. Kidney Issues:

- Kidney Disease: Kidney disease can interfere with the body's ability to rid itself of Viagra. To ensure your safety and the effectiveness of the medication, your healthcare provider may need to change the dosage of Viagra if you have kidney impairment.

- Dialysis: It's important to discuss the use of Viagra with your healthcare provider in order to determine the proper dosage considerations for people who are on dialysis.

When considering Viagra, it is crucial to have an open and sincere conversation with your doctor about the condition of your kidneys and liver. Your doctor can evaluate the severity of your liver or kidney issues and provide the best treatment options based on your unique situation. To reduce any risks, they might recommend different therapies or change the Viagra dosage.

Never use Viagra or self-adjust the dosage without first consulting a healthcare professional, especially if you have liver or kidney issues. Their advice is essential to ensuring the medication is used safely and effectively while taking into account your unique medical condition.

PROBLEMS WITH BLEEDING

It's important to use caution when thinking about using Viagra (sildenafil) if you have a history of bleeding issues or are currently experiencing bleeding issues. Viagra may interact with some medications or medical conditions that cause bleeding and affect blood clotting. Here are some crucial things to remember

Bleeding Disorders: It's important to let your doctor know if you have a known bleeding disorder, such as haemophilia or von Willebrand disease, or if you exhibit unusual bleeding tendencies. Viagra may make people with these conditions more likely to bleed.

Anticoagulants and Antiplatelet Drugs: Drugs that affect blood clotting, such as anticoagulants like warfarin and antiplatelet drugs like aspirin or clopidogrel, may interact with Viagra. When these drugs are taken together with Viagra, bleeding risk increases. In order to assess potential interactions, your healthcare provider should be informed of every medication you are taking.

It's important to be aware that one of the side effects of Viagra is priapism, which is a prolonged and painful erection. This side effect is unrelated to bleeding disorders. If priapism happens, it might result in complications, such as blood flow problems and tissue damage. Seek emergency medical help if you experience priapism.

Bleeding Events: It's important to let your doctor know before taking Viagra if you recently had surgery or sustained a significant injury that caused bleeding.

Always have a thorough conversation about your medical history, including any bleeding disorders or recent bleeding events, with your healthcare provider before taking Viagra. They can evaluate your particular circumstance and offer advice regarding whether Viagra is safe for you or if you should consider alternative treatments. Due to the potential risks of bleeding problems, they may occasionally advise against using Viagra.

CANCERS OF THE BLOND

It appears that your question contains a typographical error. I take it that you're referring to blood-related cancers. Leukaemia, lymphoma, and myeloma are the three main types of blood-related cancers. Here is a quick synopsis of each:

1. Leukaemia: A form of cancer that affects the bone

marrow and blood is known as leukaemia. It causes the body to overproduce abnormal white blood cells, which prevents the body from creating healthy blood cells. Acute lymphoblastic leukaemia (ALL), acute myeloid leukaemia (AML), chronic lymphocytic leukaemia (CLL), and chronic myeloid leukaemia (CML) are just a few of the subtypes of leukaemia that can be acute or chronic.

2. Lymphoma: Lymphoma is a type of cancer that affects the immune system's lymphatic system. When lymphocytes, a type of white blood cell, develop cancer, it happens. Hodgkin lymphoma (HL) and non-Hodgkin lymphoma (NHL) are the two main types of lymphoma. NHL is a diverse group of diseases with many subtypes.

3. Multiple myeloma, also known as myeloma, is a form of cancer that develops from plasma cells. White blood cells called plasma cells produce antibodies. Malignant plasma cells build up in the bone marrow in multiple myeloma, causing complications like bone pain, anaemia, and kidney problems.

It's critical to realise that these conditions are complicated illnesses with a wide range of subtypes and variations. The specific type and stage of a blood-related cancer can have a significant impact on treatment options and outcomes. It is essential to speak with a healthcare provider who can make a proper diagnosis, go over treatment options, and offer support if you or someone you know may have a blood-related cancer. The prognosis for many bloodrelated cancers can be significantly improved with early detection and appropriate treatment.

DEFICIENCIES IN BLOOD CELLS

Blood cell shortages can cause a variety of illnesses and conditions. Red blood cells (RBCs), white blood cells (WBCs), and platelets are the three main cell types that make up blood. Each type of blood cell performs a particular function in the body, and deficiencies in any one of these blood cell types can cause a variety of diseases. Following are some typical blood cell deficiencies and the corresponding conditions:

1. Lack of Red Blood Cells (RBCs)

- Anaemia is a condition marked by a lack of red blood cells (RBCs) or a reduction in haemoglobin, the protein that carries oxygen in the blood. Hemolytic anaemia, irondeficiency anaemia, and vitamin-deficiency anaemia are common forms of anaemia.

2. Lack of White Blood Cells (WBC):

- Leukopenia: Leukopenia is a condition where the blood's WBC count is abnormally low. Numerous factors, such as viral infections, chemotherapy, and specific medications, can cause it. An elevated risk of infections can result from a low WBC count.

3. Low blood platelet count

- Thrombocytopenia, is a condition that affects the blood. A lack of platelets can increase the risk of bleeding and facilitate easy bruising because platelets are essential for blood clotting.

4. Bone Marrow Conditions:

- Multiple types of blood cell deficiencies can result from diseases of the bone marrow, which produces blood cells. Aplastic anaemia and myelodysplastic syndromes (MDS) are two conditions that can have an impact on how much RBC, WBC, and platelet production occurs.

5. Hemoglobinopathies:

- Genetic conditions known as hemoglobinopathies affect the production or structure of haemoglobin, the oxygencarrying protein in RBCs.

    Hemoglobinopathies include diseases like sickle cell anaemia and thalassemia.

6. Autoimmune Conditions:

- RBCs or other blood cells may come under attack and destruction by the immune system as a result of some autoimmune disorders, such as autoimmune hemolytic anaemia.

The specific condition and underlying cause will determine the best course of treatment for blood cell deficiencies. It might entail dietary adjustments, nutritional supplements, drugs, blood transfusions, bone marrow transplants, or other treatments. It's crucial to see a doctor for a proper diagnosis and appropriate treatment if you suspect you have a blood cell deficiency or exhibit symptoms associated with these conditions. The quality of life for those with these disorders can be significantly increased with early detection and treatment.

RISK FACTORS OF HEART DISEASE

Two prevalent and serious medical conditions that affect the cardiovascular system are heart disease and stroke. They have some similar risk factors and mechanisms, but they also differ in certain ways. Let's go over each risk factor's mechanism in detail:

1. Heart Disease Risk Factors:

High blood pressure, or hypertension, puts additional strain on the heart and blood vessels and raises the risk of heart disease.

High LDL (low-density lipoprotein) cholesterol levels can cause atherosclerosis, which is a condition that restricts blood flow through the arteries.

Smoking: Smoking harms blood vessels, reduces the amount of oxygen delivered to the heart, and speeds up the development of blood clots.

Diabetes: Due to their elevated blood sugar levels, people with diabetes are more likely to develop heart disease. glucose levels and related metabolic problems.

Obesity: Carrying around too much body weight increases the risk of developing diabetes and high blood pressure, two conditions that are associated with heart disease.

Family History: If you have a history of heart disease in your family, your risk is higher.

Physical inactivity: Obesity and other risk factors can worsen if a person doesn't regularly exercise.

Unhealthy Diet: Heart disease can be exacerbated by a diet high in salt, added sugars, and saturated and trans fats.

Chronic stress: Through a number of mechanisms, such as high blood pressure and unhealthy coping mechanisms like overeating, chronic stress may increase the risk of heart disease.

2. Stroke Risk Factors:

High blood pressure: Both heart disease and stroke have a significant risk factor associated with high blood pressure. It might cause blood to become less strong vessels in the brain, making ruptures more likely.

Atrial Fibrillation (AFib): AFib is an irregular heartbeat that can cause blood clots to form in the heart. These blood clots may then travel to the brain and cause a stroke.

High Cholesterol: Elevated cholesterol levels can help the carotid arteries, which carry blood to the brain, develop atherosclerosis. A plaque that ruptures or obstructs blood flow to the brain can cause atherosclerosis to result in a stroke.

Smoking: Smoking increases the risk of developing heart disease and helps blood clots form, which can lead to ischemic strokes.

Diabetes: Due to its effects on the brain's blood vessels and blood pressure, diabetes raises the risk of stroke.

Obesity: Being obese or overweight is connected to a higher risk of stroke.

Physical inactivity: Obesity and other stroke risk factors can result from a lack of exercise.

Heavy drinking raises blood pressure and puts people at risk for hemorrhagic strokes, which are brought on by brain bleeding.

Drug Abuse: Cocaine and other recreational drugs can increase the risk of stroke.

Mechanisms:

The gradual accumulation of plaque (atherosclerosis) in the coronary arteries, which reduces blood flow to the heart, is a common symptom of heart disease. Angina (chest pain) or heart attacks (myocardial infarction) may result from this.

Stroke: Strokes can be ischemic, which are brought on by a blocked blood vessel in the brain, or hemorrhagic, which are brought on by brain bleeding. Ischemic strokes are more frequent and may be brought on by brain artery atherosclerosis or blood clots. Strokes that haemorrhage frequently have blood vessel walls that are weak and rupture.

ULCER'S IN THE ESOPHAGEAL

Both conditions have potentially fatal or severely disabling effects. To manage risk factors, preventive measures include dietary adjustments, medication, and medical interventions. To monitor and manage your cardiovascular health, it is crucial to seek the advice of healthcare professionals and to have regular checkups.

Esophageal ulcers, also known as esophageal ulcers, are open sores or lesions that form on the esophageal lining. The muscular tube that connects the throat to the stomach is called the oesophagus, and it has the main job of carrying food and liquids from the mouth to the stomach.

Esophageal ulcers may be linked to underlying medical conditions and can result in discomfort, pain, and a variety of other symptoms. We will look at the causes, symptoms, diagnosis, and treatment of esophageal ulcers in this article.

ESOPHAGEAL ULCERS' CAUSES

Gastroesophageal Reflux Disease (GERD): Chronic acid reflux, which happens when stomach acid flows back into the oesophagus, is one of the most frequent causes of esophageal ulcers. prolonged stomach acid exposure can cause ulcers to form and the esophageal lining to deteriorate.

Esophageal ulcers can occasionally be caused by infections like the herpes simplex virus or candidiasis (a fungal infection).

Medication: If taken improperly, some medications, particularly non-steroidal anti-inflammatory drugs (NSAIDs) or bisphosphonates, can cause esophageal irritation and ulceration.

Chemical Ingestion: The esophageal lining can suffer severe damage from swallowing corrosive substances, which can result in the development of ulcers.

Radiation Therapy: Esophageal ulcers can form as a side effect in patients receiving radiation therapy for conditions like lung cancer.

Esophageal Ulcer Symptoms

It is one of the most typical symptoms to experience chest pain. The pain is frequently described as burning and could be angina or heartburn.

Dysphagia, difficulty swallowing can happen as the oesophagus narrows due to the ulcers.

Heartburn: Esophageal ulcers may be present if the heartburn is frequent or severe.

Backflow of stomach contents into the mouth or throat is referred to as regurgitation.

Some people may experience nausea and vomiting, especially right after eating.

In severe cases, esophageal ulcers can result in bleeding, which can show up as bloody vomiting or tarry, dark stools.

Diagnosis:

Typically, esophageal ulcers are diagnosed through a combination of physical examination, medical history, and diagnostic tests, such as:

Endoscopy: To visually inspect the oesophagus and confirm the presence of ulcers, a small, flexible tube with a camera is inserted through the mouth.

Biopsy: Tissue samples may be collected during endoscopy in order to conduct a biopsy in order to rule out infections or cancer.

The term "barium swallow" is a specialised X-ray that can detect any esophageal abnormalities. pH monitoring: A 24hour period of pH monitoring may be used to evaluate acid reflux.

Treatment:

The cause and severity of esophageal ulcers determine how to treat them. Typical methods include:

Proton pump inhibitors (PPIs) and H2-receptor blockers are medications that can lessen stomach acid production and aid in the healing of ulcers.

Antifungal or antiviral medications will be prescribed if infections are the root cause.

Pain management: Prescription or over-the-counter painkillers can help with discomfort.

Lifestyle Modifications: It's frequently advised to change one's diet and way of life to lessen the triggers that cause acid reflux.

Surgery may be required in rare circumstances to treat severe ulcers or to treat side effects like bleeding or strictures.

It is crucial to deal with the esophageal ulcers and adhere to medical advice from a provider for efficient management and recurrence prevention. Strictures and Barrett's oesophagus, a precancerous condition, are just two of the serious complications that untreated ulcers can cause. It is essential to seek immediate medical attention if you experience any signs of esophageal ulcers so that you can be properly diagnosed and treated. It is challenging to breathe when you have asthma, a chronic respiratory condition that affects the lungs' airways. It can result in a variety of symptoms, with individual severity varying. Typical asthmatic signs include:

Shortness of Breath: Asthmatics frequently have trouble breathing, particularly when exhaling. This might make you feel out of breath.

Wheezing: When breathing, a high-pitched whistling sound is made. It is a defining symptom of asthma and is typically heard during exhalation.

Coughing: A common asthma symptom, especially at night or in the early morning, is a persistent, occasionally dry cough.

Chest Tightness: A common asthmatic symptom that can be painful or uncomfortable is a feeling of pressure or tightness in the chest.

Increased Mucus Production: Asthma can lead to airway inflammation and excessive mucus production, which can further impede airflow.

Exercise-induced bronchoconstriction (EIB), which causes asthma symptoms in some people when they exercise, can cause coughing or wheezing.

Nocturnal (nighttime) symptoms of asthma are frequent and can cause sleep disturbances, making it challenging to get a good night's sleep.

Asthma symptoms can range from mild to severe, and they can

be brought on or made worse by a number of things, such as allergens, respiratory infections, cold air, smoke, and stress. With periods of exacerbation (asthma attacks) and remission, asthma symptoms can fluctuate. Extremely difficult breathing is a common symptom of severe asthma symptoms, which may be a medical emergency and call for immediate care.

Proper Asthma management involves creating an asthma action plan with the help of a healthcare professional, which frequently entails using drugs like bronchodilators and inhaled corticosteroids to control and prevent symptoms. In order to effectively manage the condition, lifestyle changes are also essential. These include recognising and avoiding asthma triggers. Continual follow-up with a medical professional is necessary to modify treatment regimens and guarantee that asthma is well-controlled. It's crucial to seek medical advice if you or someone you know has asthma symptoms so that the condition can be properly assessed, diagnosed, and managed.

Interactions of Ashwagandha and Viagra

Withania somnifera, an adaptogenic herb, has long been used in Ayurvedic medicine for a number of health benefits, including lowering stress and enhancing general wellbeing. Viagra (sildenafil), on the other hand, is a drug that treats erectile dysfunction by boosting blood flow to the penis. While each substance has potential advantages on its own, combining them can cause interactions and is not recommended. Regarding possible interactions between Ashwagandha and Viagra, keep the following in mind:

Effects on Blood Pressure: Both Ashwagandha and Viagra may have mild effects on blood pressure. Combining drugs that have hypotensive effects could cause a greater drop in blood pressure, which could have negative effects like lightheadedness or fainting. If you use an antihypertensive medication This interaction may be particularly problematic for those taking medications.

Vasodilation: Ashwagandha may have a mild vasodilatory effect, similar to how Viagra works by widening blood vessels. Combining the two might have an overly dramatic effect and possibly lower blood pressure.

Cardiac Effects: Although the magnitude of this effect is not well known, ashwagandha may have some effect on heart function. By raising heart rate, viagra can also impact heart health. Combining these substances may result in heart rhythm irregularities or other cardiac problems.

Individual Reactions: Medications and herbal supplements can cause different reactions in different people. Depending on individual factors like general health, sensitivity to medications, and dosage, what may be a mild interaction for one person may be more severe for another.

Engage a Healthcare Provider: It's crucial to speak with a doctor before combining any supplements or medications, particularly those for erectile dysfunction, with herbal remedies like Ashwagandha. If it is secure and suitable for your particular circumstance, they can advise you on that.

Unless specifically instructed otherwise by a healthcare provider, it is generally advised to avoid taking Ashwagandha and Viagra together. It's important to discuss treatment options with your healthcare provider if you want to address problems with erectile dysfunction in order to choose the best course of action. Based on your medical background and unique requirements, they can offer tailored advice. Furthermore, if you are already taking medications for a health condition, it's crucial to let your doctor know about any herbal supplements you are taking into account to prevent potential interactions and guarantee your safety.

Is it safe to take Viagra with statins? While statins are a class of medications used to lower cholesterol levels, Viagra (sildenafil) is a drug that is typically prescribed to treat erectile dysfunction. There is typically no direct pharmacological interaction between Viagra and statins because they each have unique mechanisms of action. However, it's critical to think about the possible side effects and safety of taking Viagra with statins, especially if you're thinking about doing so.

1. Effects on Blood Pressure: It's known that Viagra has a mild hypotensive effect, which means it can lower blood pressure. Statins, however, have no direct impact on blood pressure. Together, they may cause a more noticeable drop in blood pressure, which may result in fainting, lightheadedness, or dizziness, especially when getting out of a chair. sitting or lying down. If you already have blood pressure problems, it is crucial to take this into account.

Statins are mainly used to lower cholesterol levels, which lowers the risk of cardiovascular events like heart attacks and strokes.

2. Cardiovascular Effects. Viagra can have some indirect effects on the cardiovascular system by increasing blood flow to the penis. Combining these drugs may put more stress on the heart. Before taking Viagra with statins, talk to your doctor if you have a history of heart issues or are at risk for cardiovascular disease.

3. Liver Function: Statins may affect the liver enzymes that are crucial for the metabolization of medications. The liver also plays a major role in the metabolism of viagra. Combining the two might have an impact on the processing of these substances by the liver. It is wise to speak with a healthcare provider if you have liver problems or are taking any medications that may affect how well your liver functions.

4. Individual Variation: Reactions to drugs and drug combinations can differ depending on the individual. What is risk-free for one person may have negative side effects or risks for another. Therefore, it's crucial to consult a doctor before taking Viagra and statins to assess your unique medical history and any possible risks.

5. Speak with a Healthcare Professional: Each individual case should be examined to determine the safety of taking

Viagra with statins. They can assess your general health, current medications, and particular risk factors to offer you individualised advice. Transparency in everything is crucial the prescription drugs and dietary supplements you are taking to protect your health.

6. Alternatives and Lifestyle Changes: Your healthcare provider can look into alternative treatments or lifestyle changes to allay your concerns if you're thinking about taking Viagra for erectile dysfunction but are worried about possible interactions with statins. A heart-healthy diet, regular exercise, and quitting smoking are all lifestyle changes that can improve cardiovascular health and possibly lessen the need for drugs like statins.

Despite the fact that there is no direct pharmacological interaction between Viagra and statins, it is still important to take into account any possible side effects on liver function, blood pressure, and the cardiovascular system. A healthcare professional should evaluate the safety of such a combination while taking into account your unique circumstances health history, medication use, and particular requirements. Making decisions about the combination of these medications or looking for alternative treatments for your health issues requires open communication with your healthcare provider There are no known significant direct interactions between omeprazole and viagra (sildenafil), two medications with distinct goals and modes of action. There are a few things to keep in mind, though, just like with any drug combination:

Metabolism and Absorption: Omeprazole is a proton pump inhibitor (PPI) that is frequently used to lessen the production of stomach acid. In the stomach, viagra is absorbed, and the liver is where it is broken down. Omeprazole may alter the pH of the stomach, which may affect how well Viagra is absorbed. Although there are no well-established interactions, taking Viagra with a PPI might theoretically have some impact on how well it is absorbed.

Effects on the Digestive System: Some people who take Viagra may experience gastrointestinal side effects like indigestion and heartburn. Omeprazole is frequently recommended to treat both acid reflux and heartburn. Omeprazole may help with the symptoms of stomach discomfort that may occur while taking Viagra.

Individual Reactions: People respond to medications differently, and what one person tolerates well may have different effects on another. It's crucial to keep an eye out for any negative side effects when combining medications.

Consult a Healthcare Professional: It is advised to speak with a healthcare professional who is familiar with your medical history, current medications, and any particular health issues before taking both medications simultaneously. They can offer tailored advice on the security of this pairing and whether any modifications are required.

In general, significant interactions or negative effects are not frequently linked to the use of Viagra and Omeprazole together. Nevertheless, as with any medication combination, particular circumstances and Particular health issues should be taken into account. You must keep lines of communication open with your healthcare provider and let them know about all the prescription drugs and dietary supplements you are taking. They can evaluate your particular circumstance and offer advice to ensure your safety and treatment effectiveness.

CHAPTER FIVE

FREQUENTLY ASK QUESTION

I'm Allergic to Claritin and Sudafed. Can I still Take Viagra? Do blood thinners like Warfarin or Xarelto interact with Viagra?

If you experience allergic reactions to both Sudafed and Claritin, it's essential to be cautious when considering any new medication, including Viagra (sildenafil). Allergic reactions can vary in severity and may be caused by different ingredients or components in the medications. It's important to discuss your allergies and specific symptoms with a healthcare provider before starting any new medication, including Viagra.

Regarding interactions with blood thinners like Warfarin and Xarelto:

1. Warfarin: Viagra can potentially interact with warfarin. Both medications affect blood clotting, and combining them may increase the risk of bleeding. Your healthcare provider will need to carefully monitor your blood clotting times and adjust the doses of these medications accordingly.

2. Xarelto: Viagra is generally considered safe to use with Xarelto. There are no known significant drug interactions between Xarelto and Viagra. However, individual responses can vary, so it's essential to communicate any new medications or changes in your treatment regimen with your healthcare provider.

In summary, if you have allergies to Sudafed and Claritin, it's essential to discuss your allergies and potential options with a healthcare provider before considering Viagra or any other medication. Additionally, if you are taking blood thinners like Warfarin or Xarelto, it's crucial to inform your healthcare provider of any new medications you plan to take to ensure there are no adverse interactions and that your treatment remains safe and effective. Always consult with a healthcare professional for personalized guidance based on your specific health needs and conditions

How long does it take for Female Viagra to begin to work?

The U.S. Food and Drug Administration (FDA) has approved the use of female Viagra, also referred to as flibanserin (brand name Addyi), to treat premenopausal women with hypoactive sexual desire disorder (HSDD). Flibanserin does not function the same way as traditional Viagra (sildenafil), which is used to treat erectile dysfunction in males, and does not directly increase blood flow to genital areas. Instead, it has an impact on brain neurotransmitters that can affect sexual desire. To reap the full rewards, allow 4–8 weeks. It's important to realise, though, that not all HSDD-afflicted women will benefit from this treatment, and that each person will experience this medication differently.

Is it possible to buy Female Viagra without a prescription?

No, most nations, including the United States, require a prescription to buy Female Viagra (flibanserin). Only a healthcare professional who has examined your medical history and determined that it is an appropriate course of treatment for your condition should prescribe and oversee the use of the prescription drug flibanserin. This is due to the fact that the medication may cause side effects and/or possible drug interactions, making it crucial for a trained healthcare professional to assess your eligibility for treatment.

It's crucial to speak with a healthcare provider if you believe you may have HSDD or are experiencing sexual desire concerns. They can provide a proper evaluation, discuss treatment options, and prescribe medications when appropriate. Self-medication or purchasing prescription drugs without a prescription can be unsafe and is not advisable. Always follow the guidance of a qualified healthcare professional when considering treatment options for medical conditions like HSDD

Exist female Viagra alternatives?

For the treatment of hypoactive sexual desire disorder (HSDD) or other sexual health issues in women, Female Viagra (flibanserin) has substitutes and alternatives. Since the underlying causes of issues with sexual desire can differ from person to person, it's important to speak with a healthcare professional to determine the best course of action for your particular needs. The following are some options and strategies to think about:

Sex therapy or counselling with a licenced therapist or counsellor can be very successful in addressing issues with sexual desire and intimacy. These treatments can assist you in discovering the underlying causes of your issues, enhancing your relationship's communication, and creating plans to increase desire and sexual satisfaction.

Changes in Lifestyle: Lifestyle choices frequently have an impact on sexual desire. A healthy lifestyle, which includes regular exercise, a balanced diet, stress management, and enough sleep, can have a positive impact on one's sexual desire as well as general wellbeing.

Relationship counselling: Sexual desire can be significantly impacted by relationship problems. When it comes to addressing communication issues, conflicts, and emotional barriers that affect sexual intimacy, couples counselling or relationship therapy may be helpful.

Hormone therapy: For some women, a lack of sexual desire may be caused by hormonal imbalances, such as low levels of oestrogen or testosterone. A healthcare professional may advise hormone replacement therapy in such circumstances.

Off-Label Drugs: If medical professionals think certain drugs may be effective despite not being specifically approved for HSDD, they may prescribe them. These may consist of drugs like bupropion, which is used occasionally to address issues with sex desire.

Products sold over the counter: Some over-the-counter items, like lubricants, gels, and supplements, are positioned as tools to increase sexual desire. Their effectiveness can vary, though, and it's important to exercise caution when using them because they might not have a solid scientific foundation.

Low-dose vaginal oestrogen treatments may be prescribed for postmenopausal women who are experiencing dryness and discomfort in their vagina. These might increase sexual interest and comfort.

Psychoeducation: It can be useful to learn about sexual well-being, desire, and the variables that affect it. To address issues with sexual desire, there are numerous educational tools available, including books, websites, and online programmes.

To determine the most effective treatment, it's critical to have an open and honest discussion with a healthcare provider. suitable strategy for your particular situation. They can carry out a thorough evaluation and go over the advantages and disadvantages of various treatments. Keep in mind that there may be different treatment options available, and what works best for one person may not be the best choice for another. Finding a tailored strategy that responds to your particular needs and concerns is the aim.

Are there alternatives to Female Viagra?

In order to address low sexual desire in women, there are alternatives to Female Viagra (flibanserin). Among these options are behavioural therapy, relationship counselling, lifestyle modifications, hormonal therapy for hormonal imbalances, off-label drugs like bupropion, over-thecounter items, vaginal oestrogen for postmenopausal discomfort, and psychoeducation.

The best option will depend on the specifics of each case as well as the underlying factors that cause low sexual desire. The best and most efficient course of action for every person's particular needs and concerns must be determined in consultation with a healthcare professional

Can a girl who is 18 years old take female viagra?

Female Viagra (flibanserin) is approved to treat premenopausal women with hypoactive sexual desire disorder (HSDD). Teenagers and those under the age of 18 are not typically prescribed it. Sexual desire varies greatly from person to person, so a healthcare professional should be cautious when diagnosing HSDD. It's important to take into account any potential underlying causes, such as emotional, relationship, or lifestyle factors, for younger people who are having issues with their sexual desire. To investigate the causes of low desire and develop appropriate strategies or treatments suited to the individual's particular needs, open communication with a healthcare professional or counsellor is crucial.

Female Viagra: Is it dangerous?

The drug flibanserin, also known as female viagra, can indeed cause adverse reactions. Drowsiness, low blood pressure, and dizziness are typical side effects. These negative effects might be exacerbated by interactions with drugs and alcohol. Due to the possibility of making these conditions worse, it is also not advised for people with liver disease or a history of depression. The medication might have an adverse effect on some people. As a result, it's crucial to speak with a healthcare professional before using Female Viagra in order to assess its suitability for your particular needs and to go over the potential advantages, risks, and alternatives.

Are Viagra dosages for men and women different?

Yes, the way that Viagra (sildenafil) works for men and women is different. Viagra has a unique mechanism of action, despite the fact that it is primarily used to treat erectile dysfunction in men by boosting blood flow to the penis. Contrarily, Female Viagra (flibanserin) works by altering brain neurotransmitters to address low sexual desire in premenopausal women. These drugs are not interchangeable and each one targets a different aspect of sexual function. Female Viagra is not intended for use by men and Viagra for men is not approved for use in women. Individual responses and needs with regard to sexual health may differ, so it's crucial to speak with a healthcare professional for specific advice.

There hasn't been much research done on how Female Viagra (flibanserin) affects transgender people who transition from male to female. Although it's primarily designed for cisgender women, some trans people have looked into using this medication to address issues with sexual desire. Individual differences in potential effects as well as hormonal and physiological influences may exist. It's critical to speak with a qualified healthcare professional with experience in transgender healthcare to discuss the potential advantages, risks, and alternatives while taking into account each person's particular circumstances. Self-medication can be dangerous, and expert guidance is essential to guarantee safety and effectiveness.

What medications are there to increase female libido?

In order to address low female libido or sexual desire, the following medications and treatments may be taken into consideration:

An FDA-approved treatment for premenopausal women with hypoactive sexual desire disorder (HSDD) is female Viagra (flibanserin).

Hormone Replacement Therapy (HRT) can treat hormonal

imbalances that have an impact on libido in postmenopausal women.

Bupropion: This antidepressant has the potential to increase sexual desire when used off-label.

Topical oestrogen: For postmenopausal women, a topical application of low-dose oestrogen can reduce vaginal discomfort and enhance libido.

Testosterone therapy may be helpful for some females who experience low libido because of hormonal problems.

These treatments should be discussed with a medical professional who can assess each patient's needs and suggest the best course of action after conducting a thorough evaluation.

ABOUT THE AUTHOR

Dr. Chris David

Dr. Chris David, MD
Gynecologist Extraordinaire

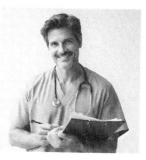

Meet Dr. Chris David, a distinguished gynaecologist renowned for his unwavering commitment to women's health. With over two decades of experience, Dr. David has been a beacon of care and compassion in the field of gynaecology. His expertise in women's reproductive health, coupled with his gentle demeanour, has earned him the trust of countless patients. Dr. David's dedication to empowering women to take charge of their health and embrace the "Lady Era" of their lives is at the heart of his practice. "My mission is to ensure every woman's journey through life is one of vitality and confidence.

Made in the USA
Monee, IL
24 November 2024

71050587R00075